Dyslexia and English

BDA/Fulton Dyslexia Series
Series editors Lindsay Peer CBE and Gavin Reid

Dyslexia and English

Elizabeth Turner and Jayne Pughe

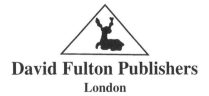

David Fulton Publishers

London

David Fulton Publishers Ltd
The Chiswick Centre, 414 Chiswick High Road, London W4 5TF

www.fultonpublishers.co.uk

First published in Great Britain in 2003 by David Fulton Publishers
10 9 8 7 6 5 4 3 2

Note: The right of Elizabeth Turner and Jayne Pughe to be identified
as the authors of this work has been asserted by them in accordance
with the Copyright, Designs and Patents Act 1988.

David Fulton Publishers is a division of Granada Learning Limited,
part of Granada plc.

British Library Cataloguing in Publication Data
A catalogue record for this book is available from the British
Library.

ISBN 1 85346 967 X

Typeset by Pracharak Technologies (P) Ltd, Madras, India
Printed and bound in Great Britain by Ashford Colour Press Ltd,
Gosport, Hants

Contents

Foreword

We are delighted to write this foreword for *Dyslexia and English*. This book is one of the books in the innovative Dyslexia Inclusion series. The aim of the series is to help subject teachers to understand the needs of learners with dyslexia in each of the different subject areas. In that way dyslexic learners will have their entitlement to a full curriculum realised.

This book by Elizabeth Turner and Jayne Pughe will go a long way towards achieving that aim. Interestingly, English is a subject that can be enjoyed by learners with dyslexia, and many select English as a subject for further and higher education. At the same time, of course, the difficulties with reading, structure, grammar and sometimes written expression can often make English a subject to dread. This is unfortunate, as the skills in creativity often noted in learners with dyslexia can lead to imaginative and vividly descriptive writing. But first there is a hurdle to overcome.

The authors of this book have ensured that the subject is well covered. They look at not only the difficulties with English grammar and preparing for examinations, but also important issues such as management and classroom environment. The book is rich in examples of practical tips for teachers, as well as structured suggestions for teaching English grammar and staff development. Their advice on dyslexia-friendly classrooms is particularly useful and, as they say, 'workspaces can become dyslexia-friendly very easily'. There is no significant financial cost to ensuring that the classroom environment is helpful for the learner with dyslexia.

But perhaps one of the most important messages to come from the book is, in the authors' own words, 'The book aims to dispel the myth that only specialist dyslexia teachers can teach dyslexic pupils successfully in the mainstream classroom. Armed with some of the ideas we have put forward we hope that the reader has gained confidence to deliver the full English curriculum in a dyslexia-friendly way.' As editors of this series we are sure that hope will become a reality, and know that if teachers of English are able to utilise some of the suggestions in this book in their daily work the skills and confidence of learners with dyslexia will be significantly enhanced.

Dr Lindsay Peer CBE
Dr Gavin Reid

Acknowledgements

We would like to thank, for their help and support, the following: all the dyslexic pupils we have had the pleasure of teaching over the years; the Headteacher and staff of Hawarden High School; Mr John Clutton, Director of Education, Libraries and Information for Flintshire.

Dedication

This book is dedicated to:

My granddaughter, Chloe Emma Turner. May she grow up to love English literature and her British heritage. E.T.

My parents Richard and Dot, who have always believed in me, and Andrew, for his patience, tolerance and above all his great support. J.P.

Chapter 1

Introduction

This book is written by two experienced practitioners who teach and support dyslexic pupils in their teaching and learning in a secondary school. It is essentially a practical book in its approach to helping pupils, their parents and mainstream teachers to overcome some of the barriers dyslexia can present in the English mainstream classroom. It is not intended to be theoretical and is based on successful practices and approaches to teaching and learning accumulated over the past thirty years. The authors strongly believe that when dyslexic pupils are taught effectively and efficiently, this has a positive effect on all pupils, and the approaches necessary to support dyslexic pupils in the English classroom are appropriate for all pupils.

> Good dyslexic teaching practice is good teaching practice. (Turner 2001)

> Inclusion means being included, being part of and having access to. (Turner 2001)

Inclusion is an entitlement. Inclusion for dyslexic pupils in the English mainstream classroom can be achieved by using a variety of strategies to support their learning. This book emphasises the importance of these strategies in the core literacy skills of reading, writing, spelling and handwriting and in the applied language and literature. Dyslexic pupils have diverse strengths and weaknesses. When we talk about tackling dyslexia we are talking about good teaching that takes account of learning styles, scaffolds development, is multisensory and is success driven. These approaches benefit all pupils.

We have written this book for the following audience: new English teachers, non-special educational needs specialist English teachers, parents and pupils themselves. We have avoided jargon but have introduced and explained key terms and concepts. This is in order to empower the reader. Knowledge about a child's special needs can often seem to be hidden behind a closed door to non-specialists because of the way 'experts' bandy terms around without explanation. In special needs departments these terms are used so often that professionals forget that they are alien to many people. There are so many acronyms that it can sometimes seem as though we are speaking and writing in a foreign language.

'Has the SENCO sent the IEP to the EP?'
'No, the ESW gave it to the ASW.'

('Has the special educational needs coordinator sent the individual education plan to the educational psychologist?'
'No, the educational social worker gave it to the ancillary support worker.')

Teaching dyslexic children and conversing with their parents can be at times a hit and miss affair without a positive, practical and sympathetic approach. The onus here is very much on the teacher to provide understanding, access and support in all aspects of pupils' teaching and learning.

Historically, English, especially the language sections, is the area where there is a great fear of failure, and is one of the most difficult dyslexic learners are challenged with in the examination system. This is because dyslexic pupils are confronted with being tested and examined in the areas where they are experiencing the most difficulty. In other words, they are being tested on their weaknesses. No wonder the word 'English' can bring with it such emotional baggage and can be loaded with connotations. 'English' conjures up accuracy in spelling, writing and reading – the things with which most dyslexic learners have experienced difficulty in their day-to-day life.

Helping dyslexic children to manoeuvre their way through the subject that often causes them the most difficulties can be traumatic. You know they need English qualifications for their next steps in life, but they may see English lessons as hour-long sessions that stretch their avoidance tactics to the limit.

This book is divided into sections that cover the English curriculum. This is in order to allow 'dippers' quick access to relevant material. We recognise all too well that time is the teacher's most precious commodity and the book aims to help, not to make even more work. Parents similarly often do not have the time, or if they are dyslexic themselves possibly the skills, needed to wade through heavyweight academic books on the subject. They need and want practical help and understanding to support their children to fulfil their learning potential. Parents want happy children who are successful and who achieve. Teachers and pupils want the same. We hope this book can be a reference book that answers some questions, gives practical tips on what has and what has not worked for us and tackles problems as they arise.

The book is based on experience, and the advice has been tried and tested. We have a combined special needs teaching experience of forty years and we look at the problems, the challenges and successes from both a teaching and a personal point of view.

Elizabeth Turner is dyslexic herself and has two children who are dyslexic and have successfully completed their education to university level (one graduating with a first class honours degree). She has set up, runs and manages a county dyslexia provision based in a secondary school since its conception in 1991. For the past eleven years she has exclusively taught dyslexic pupils in a mainstream setting, so her views are based on personal experience not only of dyslexia in the family, but also of what works and what doesn't in the teaching setting.

Jayne Pughe is an English specialist who started with little knowledge of dyslexia. Her PGCE course had covered special needs briefly and provided the opportunity to work with experienced practitioners in her placement schools. Working with and learning from excellent teachers has been the basis of her success with dyslexic pupils.

Chapter 2

Dealing with Dyslexia in the English Department

Reading

> For the public at large, the term Dyslexia is usually restricted to reading difficulties. (West 1991: 79)

There is a popular misconception among laypeople that being dyslexic means that you cannot read, or have great difficulty with reading. Furthermore, people often believe that letters and words somehow appear written or spoken in the wrong order. Dyslexia has been and still is the butt of many jokes and black humour, which perpetuates this myth. DYSLEXIA RULES KO is an example of the type of humour and the sort of misunderstanding that is circulating and often misleads the general population. Having said that, we will appear to contradict ourselves by saying that there are and will be dyslexic pupils who do experience severe reading difficulties and will always have some problems with mastering the mechanics of reading. However, the important point here is that these dyslexic pupils are the minority and not the majority. We consider dyslexia to be on a continuum – that is, you can be dyslexic from a mild level through to moderate and severe levels. We would expect the severe reading difficulties to appear at the severe end of the continuum and vice versa.

There are many dyslexic learners who have mastered the mechanics of reading successfully and to all appearances are no

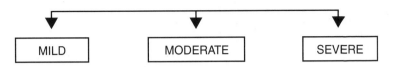

Figure 2.1 A Continuum of Dyslexia

different from their non-dyslexic peers when it comes to reading ability. However, what we have noticed from our hands-on teaching with dyslexic youngsters is that although fluent dyslexic readers can read competently and in many instances with great skill, frequently they read at a slower rate than their non-dyslexic counterparts. It takes them longer to read in detail and to comprehend what they have read. In other words, these are the pupils who read slowly and frequently lose meaning in the process. They appear at times to 'bark at print' and may have difficulty recognising and adapting their reading style to the reading purpose. Do not presume that these pupils know, as if by some osmotic process, the most appropriate and efficient reading method to use for a given task. They need to be taught explicitly the skill of choosing which reading method best suits a task and need to be able to identify the purpose and adapt their reading style to it.

Supporting students means teaching them exactly what type of reading to use and giving them practice in that skill. (Turner 2001: 65)

Detailed reading

Detailed reading, as the name suggests, means just that – attention to detail. Every word must be read carefully so that there is no ambiguity. Examination questions, instructions and legal contracts are the best examples of the type of reading material that requires this technique. All pupils would benefit from being taught when detailed reading is needed and why. What might seem obvious to you as a parent or teacher may not seem so obvious to the pupil, who may be thinking, learning and seeing things in their mind's eye in a different way. A multisensory approach with an emphasis on the kinaesthetic and visual channels would be one of the best ways to approach this. We often use the test shown in Figure 2.3 as a starting point to illustrate the importance of following test instructions. Pupils get very annoyed when they fall into the trap of not reading carefully. By not following the written instructions in this test to the letter, they waste their own time!

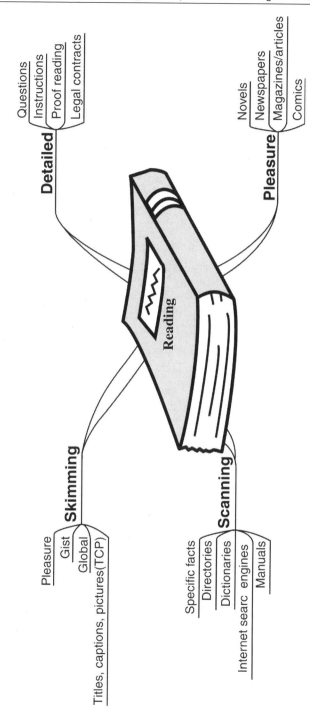

Detailed
- Questions
- Instructions
- Proof reading
- Legal contracts

Pleasure
- Novels
- Newspapers
- Magazines/articles
- Comics

Reading

Skimming
- Pleasure
- Gist
- Global
- Titles, captions, pictures(TCP)

Scanning
- Specific facts
- Directories
- Dictionaries
- Internet searc engines
- Manuals

Figure 2.2 Matching Reading Style to Purpose

Pupils are told they are having a test under strict examination conditions and the test will last five minutes. Pupils are issued with an individual question paper that is placed question side down. The invigilator starts the test and the pupils turn their paper over and complete it. At regular one-minute intervals the invigilator tells the pupils how much time is left. This is to put the pupils under time pressure. When the time is up all pupils put their pencils down. It amazes us that in a class of 30, the majority will not use a detailed reading approach when reading instructions for a 'Test on Following Instructions'. They usually only make this mistake once!

Skimming

This involves looking at the 'big' picture and using clues on the page to help to get the gist or feeling of a passage, extract or book. It is quick reading, 'skimming' over the surface of the page. It is the reading we do when we want to get an idea or overview of a written passage or piece of work. It is not involved with detail. Skimming is used to read articles in newspapers and magazines. It is used frequently when we read for pleasure. The message to get across here to the pupil is IT IS NOT NECESSARY TO READ EVERY SINGLE WORD on the page IN CERTAIN SITUATIONS. Pupils need to know it is perfectly in order and not only effective but also efficient to skim. Some pupils will need to be told this explicitly and taught this skill. Other pupils may need to be given 'permission' to use this technique. If they have struggled with reading and read laboriously, word by word, they may assume that all readers read this way and all reading material should be read in the same way. Most instructions for comprehension exercises require the pupil to read the passage through once or twice. This is often cited as the first instruction. We would argue that this is not the most effective or efficient way to attack comprehension. Our target is for maximum efficiency with minimum effort. From practical experience of teaching in secondary schools, we can say that this idea appeals to many teenagers! We teach our pupils to look for clues. They look at headings, words in bold or italic, instructions, pictures, diagrams and any summaries first. This is to gain a general impression or overview. It will give them some idea about the passage. We then direct them to the questions and encourage them to skim the

Test   **Following Instructions**

This is a timed test. You have five minutes only.

1. Read everything carefully before you begin.

2. Write your name in BLOCK letters in the left hand corner of your paper.

3. Underline your surname with a ruler.

4. Draw three small triangles and a circle in the top right hand corner.

5. Put a dot in the circle and a 'x' in each of the triangles.

6. Draw a line to join the triangles and circles.

7. Put your signature in the left-hand side bottom corner.

8. PRINT your name above your signature.

9. Draw a box around your signature and name.

10. Put a tick at each corner of this box.

11. Write 'Yes' at the top of this box and 'No' at the bottom.

12. Draw the letter E in the bottom right hand corner.

13. Put a circle around this letter.

14. In the middle of the page add 1356 + 2734.

15. Draw an oblong around the answer.

16. Shout your name out.

17. If you have got this far and carried out all the instructions above, shout YES.

18. Under the addition sum, subtract 157 from 2009.

19. Draw a rectangle around your answer and put 4 stars in each corner of it.

20. The only thing to do in this test is to write your name at the top of the page.

Figure 2.3 Following Instructions Test

passage and annotate where the answer to each question may be. We recommend the use of highlighter pens for this task. Obviously, any questions requiring inference from the passage would need to be left to a later stage after the first skimming of the entire passage is complete. This skimming gives the pupil a feel, sense or general impression of the passage. Then, and only then, do we encourage the pupil to read in greater depth and answer the questions. This technique is particularly useful to the global thinker whose preferred learning style is 'seeing' things within the context of the larger picture.

Scanning

Scanning means looking for specific facts and information on a page. This is a quick, efficient reading technique used for a particular purpose. It may seem a very obvious and easy reading skill to use but, again, many pupils find scanning initially hard, especially after they have been used to reading every single word on the page or have struggled with reading. Telephone directories, manuals, indexes, encyclopaedias and Internet search engine results are good examples of information gleaning sources that require scanning. Target or key words are used to scan the page. Pupils will need to be taught explicitly what a key word is. This is the foundation for later work on paragraph development, where key words and sentences are so important, and in the use of mind webbing for planning and revision. This is explored in more detail in Chapter 6. What we suggest may seem to you to be common sense and quite obvious. However, pupils are frequently told to use 'something' and they have no idea what that 'something' is. For example, how do you recognise a key word if you don't know what one is?

Reading for pleasure

We believe that reading is a human right and is the essence of inclusion. Being able to read and to use that skill means you have the key to a door that opens into a world of adventure, fantasy and imagination. It is the membership card to a worldwide club where all are eligible to join regardless of colour, race, creed, gender and class. This membership gives access not only to what is within the pages of a book but also to communication and knowledge. In the secondary school there is concern that, for a variety of reasons, pupils are reading less than ever – especially fiction. Motivating and encouraging pupils to read fiction,

Key Words are the ones that

UNLOCK your mind.

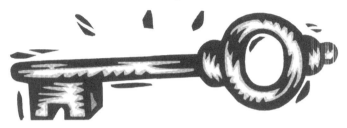

Verbs and Nouns are key words.

They are loaded with meaning

Figure 2.4 Key Words

especially teenage boys, who often are 'reluctant readers', can be a challenging task. It is important that these readers are given access to age-appropriate literature. This is because of issues of educational and social inclusion. When pupils meet their peers socially they will have the same literary experiences and background and can participate in oral discussions. One way of increasing access to literature is to provide the reluctant reader with cover-to-cover audiotapes of the book involved, at the same time giving them the hard copy to follow. For example, we use the Harry Potter books with a group of Year 8 boys backed up by the audiotapes. Based on the criteria that the boys related to reading in a positive and enjoyable way and wanted more, we judge this to be a successful technique.

Motivating reluctant readers
If it has been a struggle to reach a reading age of seven, eight or nine years, reading for pleasure will be a paradoxical term for many pupils. Reading for fun is something that other people do, not them.

Dragging themselves through textbooks and class readers that are too difficult is what they have to do. Experience has shown that this is a crucial barrier to get through for dyslexic pupils and all pupils who struggle with their reading.

For secondary school English teachers, it is often too difficult to address this need. There is so much to get through in two or three hours a week that this can inadvertently be sidelined. It is an issue that encroaches on many aspects of the pupil's personality and a teacher can often be afraid of upsetting, angering or embarrassing a pupil by encouraging him or her to read during private reading sessions instead of staring into space or annoying others. We have found a number of ways to motivate these reluctant readers.

One such motivating technique is the Reading Passport. This was devised and produced by Jayne Pughe and Debbie Smith and piloted at Hawarden High School in Flintshire, North Wales, in 1998 following an HMI inspection. At this inspection, the English department was questioned over the breadth of books that pupils read for pleasure. The inspector had seen lots of 'Goosebumps' and 'Point Horror' being read and recorded on reading logs. We had seen passports used in local libraries and adapted these examples to develop a scheme for the department. The school invested in books and some reading trolleys for classrooms. All these books were labelled to link them to the categories on the passports. The school librarian devised lists of books available to supplement some of the harder categories, such as 'Journeys' and 'Other Cultures'. As a department we established ground rules about some of the categories.

In order to give pupils clear guidelines and structure, interpretation of categories had to be explicit. The scheme has been used with Key Stage 3 pupils and has proven highly successful. It is competitive and the pupils enjoy it. 'It makes you want to read because you want to fill up your passport' (Year 10 pupil, 2003). The categories can be marked off with a pen, or for Year 7, special stickers. Merits are awarded when pupils finish a passport. They can read at home and write these books on their reading logs and therefore complete a box. If we suspect cheating, or more importantly if other pupils do, we ask for confirmation from parents in the pupil's planner.

The reading passport is used across the ability range. You cannot motivate reluctant readers by making them stand out. The passport is designed to enable all readers to get something out of it. The more able readers will be guided to make challenging choices, especially when they work through the third passport. Reluctant readers can complete passports by reading 'Quick Reads'. These are a range of readers that are short and have text that is accessible to pupils with reading ages of seven to nine years. There are some excellent books that fulfil this criterion on the market.

These books are labelled with a sticker that says 'Quick Reads'. They are available to everyone. We supplement them with county library project loans that connect to topics being studied or are of a particular genre. It is important to make sure that the 'Quick Reads' do not have any form of stigma attached to them. They must not be seen as the 'special' books for specific pupils. You should try to steer the more able but 'lazy' readers away by generating interest in particular authors, film tie-ins or reading award shortlists, such as the 'Askew's Award', 'Smarties Prize' or 'Carnegie Medal'.

The following are some of the 'Quick Reads' we recommend:

- *Spirals*, published by Stanley Thornes.

- *Sprinters*, published by Walker Books.

- *Solo Transport* and *Solo Animals*, published by Southwood Books.

- Anything in the *Livewire* series, published by Hodder & Stoughton.

- *Super Crunchies*, published by Orchard Books.

We have found that plays have helped to generate enthusiasm for reading in even the most reluctant readers. They usually start by listening in to others. We legitimised this important stage by making reluctant readers the prompt. They then start to take smaller roles when they have become familiar with the play. Plays are good value for money because if they are popular the children will perform them over and over again. For someone who is catching up with his or her peers this can provide an opportunity to listen to good models of reading. We find that it develops scanning skills when pupils are looking for their cues. Pupils listen to each other in order to follow the script. Their expression develops as they listen to each other and copy good readers. The most popular plays we use are *Impact Plays*, published by Ginn. Steve Barlow's and Steve Skidmore's plays are our pupils' favourites.

but to places deep beneath the ocean and far off into space. This

This is a passport to anywhere. Not just on earth,

passport, if used correctly, will transport you back

in time to the age of the dinosaurs or forward to the future...

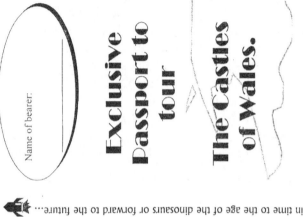

Name of bearer:

Exclusive Passport to tour

The Castles of Wales.

Figure 2.5 (i)

Don't forget to keep a record of your travels to help those who follow you! Please list and rate the books you have read on your reading log.

Here is a ratings guide to help you:

-Would not even recommend to my worst enemy!

-Good, would recommend a visit to a friend.

-Excellent! I'll go there again!

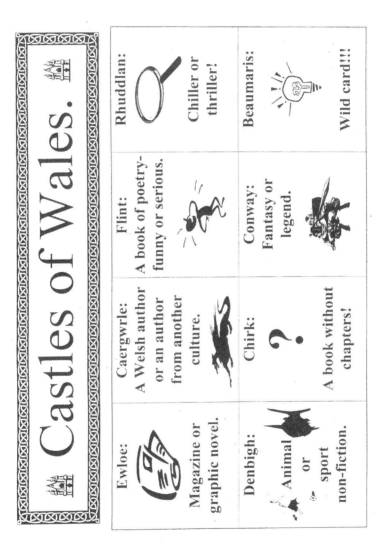

Castles of Wales.

Ewloe: Magazine or graphic novel.

Caergwrle: A Welsh author or an author from another culture.

Flint: A book of poetry— funny or serious.

Rhuddlan: Chiller or thriller!

Denbigh: Animal or sport non-fiction.

Chirk: A book without chapters!

Conway: Fantasy or legend.

Beaumaris: Wild card!!!

Figure 2.5 (ii)

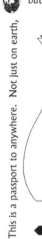

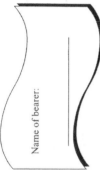

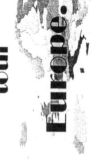

but to places deep beneath the ocean and far off into space. This

This is a passport to anywhere. Not just on earth,

Name of bearer:

Exclusive Passport to tour Europe.

passport, if used correctly, will transport you back

in time to the age of the dinosaurs or forward to the future...

Figure 2.5 (iii)

Don't forget to keep a record of your travels to help those who follow you! Please list and rate the books you have read on your reading log.

Here is a ratings guide to help you:

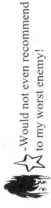

-Would not even recommend to my worst enemy!

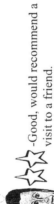

-Good, would recommend a visit to a friend.

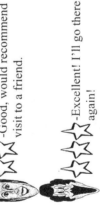

-Excellent! I'll go there again!

Devised and produced by J.L. Pughe and D. Smith. English and Performing Arts Faculty Hawarden High School.

A European Tour.

Cardiff	London	Paris	Madrid	Rome
Myths, legends or fantasy novel/ virtual reality.	Biography or autobiography.	Poetry-romance or other cultures.	Adventure or historical.	Sport fiction or animal fiction.
Vienna	Budapest	Prague	Berlin	Brussels
Fiction-teen angst or other cultures.	Chiller or thriller!	Horrible Science or Horrible Histories.	Journeys.	Wild card!!!

Figure 2.5 (iv)

This is a passport to anywhere. Not just on earth, but to places deep beneath the ocean and far off into space. This passport, if used correctly, will transport you back in time to the age of the dinosaurs or forward to the future...

Exclusive Passport to tour

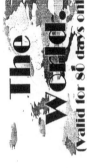

The World!
(Valid for 80 days only!)

Name of bearer:

Figure 2.5 (v)

Don't forget to keep a record of your travels, to help those who follow you! Please list and rate the books you have read on your reading log.

Here is a ratings guide to help you:

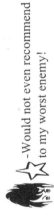
☆ -Would not even recommend to my worst enemy!

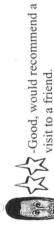
☆☆ -Good, would recommend a visit to a friend.

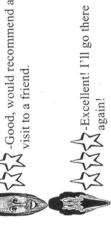
☆☆☆ -Excellent! I'll go there again!

Around the World in 80 Days.

Folkestone: Magazine or joke book.	Venice: Environmental or social issues (fact or fiction).	Athens: Weird Science or Horrible Histories.	Cairo: Biography or autobiography.	Bombay: Classic prose or poetry.
Singapore: Adventure or historical.	Hong Kong: Other cultures or teen angst.	Shanghai: Fantasy or graphic novel.	Chicago: Travelogue, fiction or non-fiction.	New York: Classic poetry or prose.
				London: Wild card!!!

Figure 2.5 (vi)

now an independent traveller. Remember you must challenge

This is your ticket to explore the universe. You are

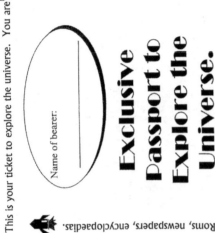

Name of bearer:

Exclusive Passport to Explore the Universe.

Subject of your quest:

yourself if you want to benefit from your quest.

Poetry, plays, novels, CD Roms, newspapers, encyclopaedias.

Don't forget to keep a record of your travels to help those who follow you! Please list and rate the books you have read on your reading log.

Explore the Universe.

You have travelled around the world and now you are free to explore the universe! This passport is difficult to complete but it will be worth it. Go on challenge yourself!

Pick a topic that you are really interested in.

Ask your English teacher for some examples to help you choose.

Select a **range** of reading materials that will help you to study this topic. The wider the range the more enjoyable the quest.

Devised and produced by J.L. Pughe and D. Smith.
English and Performing Arts Faculty Hawarden High School.

Figure 2.5 (vii)

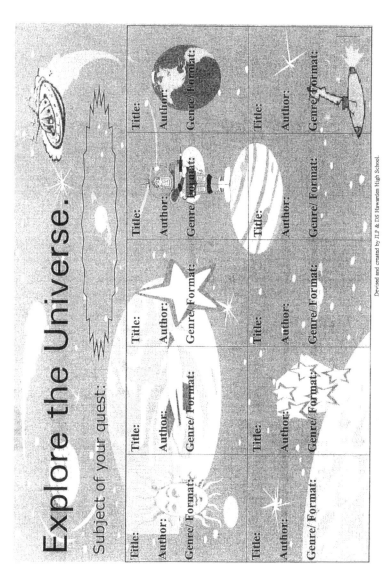

Figure 2.5 (viii)

Only you know
your limits.

These are only suggestions.
We would be delighted to hear
any other ideas.

Remember: wide
range of materials
studied =
a fantastic journey!

Good luck!

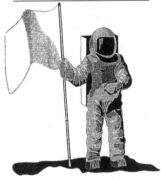

Designed and produced by
J.L.Pughe and D. Smith,
the Faculty of English and Performing Arts, Hawarden
High School.

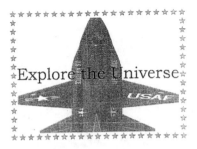

Explore the Universe

Some ideas to help you
to decide 'where' to go.

**Any topic you choose can be
explored through a range of
reading:**
poetry,
plays,
novels,
newspaper articles,
CD ROMs,
the Internet,
magazines.
encyclopaedias,
text books,
diaries,
autobiographies,
travel writing...

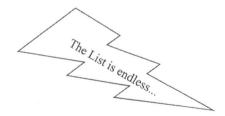

The List is endless...

Figure 2.5 (ix)

History

You could study the history of any period. Some examples are World War II, the Sixties, ancient Greece or Egypt.

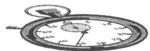

Why not study the history of the whole millennium!

You could choose to look at works that tell us things about different stages of history. Here are some ideas: Beowulf, stories from the New Testament, Chaucer, Shakespeare, Samuel Pepys' diary, Anne Frank's diary, Encarta entries on Nelson Mandela, newspaper articles about the death of Princess Diana.

Places

You could centre your search around a country or a continent.

This could be your dream holiday destination.

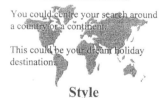

Style

You could choose to study a style e.g. poetry, drama, diaries or autobiography.

You could look at works from different countries, different periods in history or different genres.

Genre

If you enjoy a certain genre you could trace its development (the history). For example, you could trace detective stories from Edgar Alan Poe to Ruth Rendell or Sci-fi from Mary Shelley to Pratchett.

Interests

If you are mad about horses, obsessed by cars or a football fanatic then you

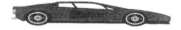

could use your interest as the basis of your study.

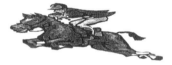

Authors

If you really like a certain author you could read one or two books by them, their autobiography, something about where they are from and then some authors who are similar to them.

Don't forget to look in 'Books for Keeps' which is kept in the library.

If any texts needed to finish a study are too difficult or too long you can read abridged versions or versions written for younger readers.

Figure 2.5 (x)

Reading for pleasure is something that links a pupil to the peer group and offers the opportunity to go on adventures together. If everyone has been to Hogwart's, Narnia and Middle Earth except you, it can be extremely frustrating. As the reading passport says, books offer 'a passport to anywhere. Not just on earth, but to places deep beneath the ocean and far off into space. This passport, if used correctly, will transport you back in time to the age of the dinosaurs or forward to the future.' Part of the pleasure of going on these 'journeys' is talking about them when you get back. We have witnessed many pupils' transformation from non-readers to readers. The difference it has made in all areas of the curriculum and the confidence it has generated are considerable.

Spelling

Difficulties mastered are opportunities won. (Winston Churchill)

One of the most difficult challenges the mainstream English teacher faces in the classroom is the question of spelling. The pupil who is articulate and bright, asks searching questions, contributes orally in a positive and intelligent manner yet has a significant difficulty in spelling accuracy presents the teacher with a dichotomy. Why cannot this bright pupil spell accurately and what can be done to help him or her in the mainstream classroom? Weakness in spelling accuracy frequently leads not only to negative assumptions being made about a pupil by responsible adults, but also to self-judgements being made by the speller himself and his peer group. Feelings of inadequacy, frustration and low self-esteem creep into an already fragile personality and often damage personal confidence levels. Spelling is therefore an emotive issue and one that brings emotional baggage with it for the dyslexic pupil. Weakness in spelling accuracy, and fear of failure and ridicule, restricts the pupil on the written page.

Spelling and reading, although interrelated, involve quite different skills. Reading is a decoding skill, where a pupil can be helped by clues to work out the word to be read. Spelling, on the other hand, is an encoding process, which involves the total recall of words, which then have to be reproduced accurately from memory. The skills a competent speller requires are:

- good visual recall of words involving accurate mental imagery;
- good auditory discrimination;
- an awareness of sound symbol correspondence.

These are the very things that are weaknesses in a dyslexic profile. Many dyslexic learners master the mechanics of reading in the early stages of their education, but accuracy in spelling is more difficult to achieve. Often spelling remains a lifelong difficulty.

Although reading has always been given more prominence than spelling, the latter in fact poses the greater problem for dyslexic children. This difficulty can continue long after the reading difficulty has been greatly improved. 'Poor spelling is usually a lifetime's embarrassment' (Pollock and Waller 1994: 39).

Frith (1981) indicates that spelling skills are directly related to the student's metalinguistic awareness – that is, the acquisition of language skills in relation to the development of language. This has important implications for English teaching. Improvements and accuracy in spelling can be helped by explicitly teaching the reasons why words are spelt the way they are to all pupils – dyslexic and non-dyslexic. Spelling becomes more predictable and logical when pupils have an understanding of how and why letters relate to each other. Instead of trying to grasp a whole word image, which relies on sequential memory, the pupil armed with this knowledge can work out what is the most probable way to spell a word. They need to use their higher-level thinking skills to help them. Pupils need to know what consonants and vowels are, their functions, the use of short vowels and how they affect the letters following them, the role of long vowels, different ways of spelling a sound and the part that syllables play in both reading and writing. Knowing about and using diacritical marks helps to illustrate the spelling/sound differences between long and short vowels, which is crucial when teaching spelling.

For competence in spelling, pupils need to have a knowledge of the alphabet and of the importance of vowels and their sounds, rhyming ability, phonemic awareness, a knowledge of segmentation, clear articulation, a legible cursive script and good visual brain imagery. These are often areas of weakness for many dyslexic learners; hence the spelling difficulties that are apparent in their written work.

25

Spelling strategies

One of the first ways of tackling spelling is to give all pupils some strategies to use. Pupils who struggle with spelling will ask for the spelling of a particular word in the classroom situation. Many teachers will give that spelling in an auditory way or write it on a piece of paper for the pupil to copy. We believe this is not an effective way of teaching the spellings of words. It may answer a need at a particular time but the dyslexic pupil, when faced with the same word again, will not have learned it efficiently and so will not remember the sequence of letters and reproduce it accurately.

All spelling strategies should embrace multisensory teaching and learning techniques. That is, any strategies used should utilise all the senses when learning.

The visual inspection technique is the LOOK, SAY, COVER, SAY, WRITE, CHECK method, which is widely used. Briefly, this requires the pupil to ask for the word, which is written down. The pupil then looks at the word carefully and says it aloud. The word is then covered up and the pupil says the word aloud again, *as it is written down from memory*. The word is then checked with the original for accuracy.

Another popular and effective strategy is the use of mnemonics to aid spelling. Most of the general population uses this technique to spell awkward words, the words we are never quite sure of, and to remember important dates and facts. The beauty of mnemonics is that they are often visually strong and colourful, utilising right hemispherical brain functioning, in which many dyslexic pupils have strengths. Mnemonics are visual pegs upon which to anchor a spelling in the mind. The most effective mnemonics are also humorous and rude. (In fact, the ruder the better in our experience!) The more personal the mnemonic, the more memorable it becomes.

Here are some mnemonics collected in the classroom and used by pupils. The list is not extensive, as personal choice plays an important role in the use of mnemonics. What works for one may or may not work for another.

- **You** are **you**ng.

- A **pie**ce of **pie**.

- Ne**cess**ary has a **cess** pit in the middle of it.

- A **bus** is **bus**y and is a good **bus**iness.

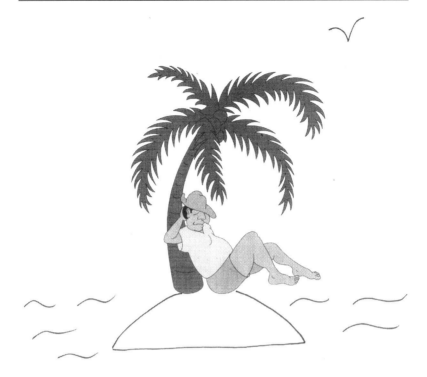

An island is Land with sea around it.

Figure 2.6 Mnemonics

- A **U** turn.

- **O U** lucky **d**uck (could, should, would).

- **E**very **G**ood **B**oy **D**eserves **F**un (the notes on the stave lines for the treble clef).

- **A**ll **C**ows **E**at **G**rass (the notes between the stave lines for the bass clef).

- **R**ichard **O**f **Y**ork **G**ave **B**attle **I**n **V**ain, or **ROY G**et **B**ack **I**n **V**an (the colours of the rainbow).

- **I** to the **end** will be your fr**iend**.

- Co**mm**i**tte**e has two **mte**.

- **Said**: **S**am **A**nd **I** **D**ance.

Another way of increasing spelling accuracy is to encourage pupils to take an interest in words themselves. Neurolinguistic programming (NLP) looks at words carefully, noticing the structure of the word, focusing on the way a word is written and asking questions about it.

- How many vowels are there in the word?
- How many ascending and descending letters are there?
- Are there any words in words going from left to right? There: the, her, he, here, ere etc.
- Is there anything unusual about the word?
- How many letters are there in the word?
- Read the letter names aloud from right to left.
- Read the letter names aloud from left to right.
- Which words have similar endings – rimes? Can the pattern be seen?

A way of encouraging an interest in words is for pupils to look at word roots, word derivations, prefixes and suffixes. The study of etymology is also a rich source of interest and provides an introduction to an awareness of words. It can explain why some words are spelt the way they are, especially the non-regular ones. When dyslexic pupils understand why words have the spellings they have, they are more likely to remember them. Pupils learn not only about the word but also how it came into our language and how our language is evolving and changing.

RIP

Another method we use for improving spelling levels with very weak spellers is one that we call RIP (Reading Improvement Programme). It is based on the successful Somerset Talking Computer Programme – with extra embellishments. We have found this to be successful in raising both spelling and reading levels within a short time scale. We use it daily for a month with three pupils whom we have assessed as having low reading and spelling levels.

Each pupil is required to carry out four tasks in any order they choose. Each task is completed within a time scale and is overseen by a learning assistant. During the course of a one-hour lesson:

- Pupils read from cards into a computer that uses voice recognition, following the instructions for the Somerset Talking Computer Programme.

- Pupils do two exercises in *tracking*, using high frequency words and sentences.

- They read Talking Books on the computer, e.g. the Famous Five series.

- They read to the teacher from a structured reading scheme.

Dictionaries

Another tool we recommend for weak spellers in the classroom is the ACE (Aurally Coded English) Spelling Dictionary. Pupils will need to be taught in a structured way to use this dictionary, but once taught, they can efficiently find words they want to spell in a very short time. In addition, there is the added bonus of being able to use the dictionary independently. There are three detailed lessons in the introduction to the dictionary that cover all the instructions pupils will need to use it successfully.

We have found this dictionary successful with dyslexic pupils, especially those who have had a history of struggling with a 'conventional' dictionary. Nevertheless, as no meanings are given in the spelling dictionary, there is a place for a conventional dictionary in school, which dyslexic learners can access. Each faculty or department in a school should devise subject-specific spelling dictionaries laid out in alphabetical or topic order. These dictionaries can target words that staff feel are necessary for accuracy in their area. In the English department, for instance, there might be a need to target high-frequency words in Year 7, but in Year 8 the emphasis on spelling accuracy may be geared towards literature or poetry, which would mean spellings related to a particular author or genre.

Multisensory structured spelling programmes

There are many excellent, well established, multisensory spelling programmes on the market (Hickey, Alpha to Omega, The Kingston Programme etc.). However, most of these are designed for individual or small-group teaching and are not appropriate for whole-class teaching without adaptation. Nevertheless there is great value in using them for reference or for ideas if you are teaching a specific spelling principle to the whole class. For example, Lucy Cowdery's *Spelling Rulebook* contains all the rules and generalisations of English spelling in a handy format. By using the rulebook, the teacher can build up an understanding of the spelling system. Good spellers frequently do not have this explicit understanding. They are able to spell the word accurately, so there is no need for them to understand why. Dyslexic pupils, on the other hand, need to understand why words are spelt in a certain way. This aids processing. It is therefore important for the teacher to understand spelling principles and rules so that this understanding can then be taught to all pupils, especially the dyslexic ones. The *Rulebook* was developed as part of the Kingston Programme (Teaching Reading through Spelling; TRTS) and is widely used. It is clear, very accessible and user friendly. In our experience no English department should be without a copy. In a survey of research on ways to improve spelling, Moseley (1994) suggests that there are many ways to teach spelling, but the most successful are the ones that combine a number of features.

> Spelling rules are a collection of short sentences that aim to give children a logical strategy that, when mastered and applied, allows them to spell hundreds of words. The advantages are that they allow the dyslexic [learner] to apply logic. (Watkins and Thomson 1990: 125)

The *Dyslexia Teaching Handbook* supports the teaching of spelling principles and rules to dyslexic pupils.

Watkins and Thomson (1990) point out that spelling principles give a simple structure and logical approach to building words, which does not rely on rote learning but uses the strength of good reasoning skills, which many dyslexic learners possess. However, a word of warning: *spelling rules or principles must not be learned in isolation – they must be used and rooted firmly in the mind, understood and transferred to all written work.*

Helpful hints for spelling development

Here are some tips to improve spelling. As a carpenter needs tools to do his job so the speller needs tools to spell accurately and a good workshop in which to operate.

- Pupils should be taught basic linguistic principles. They need to know about vowels and consonants, short and long vowels and their diacritical markings, alphabetical order and syllabication.

- The use of a highlighter is strongly recommended. Often a pupil 'knows' how to spell accurately part of a word and can easily identify the section of letters or the letter that is causing confusion or difficulty. Highlighting that area and learning using visual clues helps to reduce the overload on memory.

- The mainstream English teacher can best support dyslexic pupils in the classroom by encouraging and accepting logical spelling, if accuracy is not possible. They can help by not covering a pupil's written work with red corrections, identifying each and every spelling error. (If a pupil is weak at spelling, they already lack confidence in personal spelling ability and do not need to be further demoralised by having red marks or 'sp' scrawled all over work.) Spelling is an emotive issue. Marking, whenever and wherever possible, should be within a framework of a whole-school policy on spelling that takes account of dyslexic difficulties and gives consistency of expectation. The dyslexic pupil then has a structure within which to operate.

- There should be a whole-school policy on spelling built into the school development plan. This gives consistency across the curriculum and raises awareness, without destroying the confidence of weaker spellers.

Whole-school spelling support

The principle behind this book is that what works for dyslexic pupils works for all pupils. We have used the principles and the methodology outlined to devise materials to support all pupils. If dyslexic pupils are supported alongside everyone else, the feelings of low self-esteem and frustration are lessened.

The National Literacy Strategy recognises the need to teach spelling explicitly in a consistent and methodical way. This will benefit dyslexic learners as they progress through primary school and into secondary school. However, the Strategy does seem to encourage a one-visit approach. The amount to be taught in a term is vast. Will good spellers get even better and widen the gap?

How to Spell Well . . . Five Strategies for Spelling Success!

1. Syllables.

2. Tackle the tricky bit.

3. Use your spelling know how.

4. Mnemonics.

5. LOOK

SAY

COVER

WRITE

CHECK

Figure 2.7 Poster

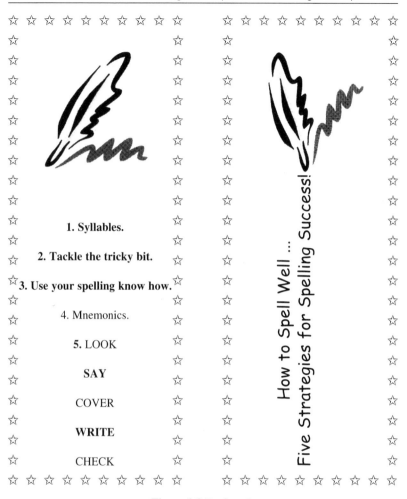

1. Syllables.

2. Tackle the tricky bit.

3. Use your spelling know how.

4. Mnemonics.

5. LOOK

SAY

COVER

WRITE

CHECK

How to Spell Well ... Five Strategies for Spelling Success!

Figure 2.8 Bookmark

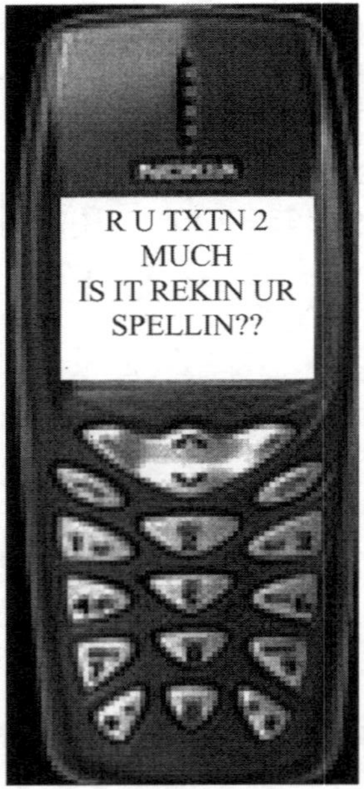

For spelling advice read on...

Figure 2.9 (i)

Tricky Words...

necessary		
occasionally		
believe		
until		
through		
quiet		
beginning		
library		
already		
knew/know		

Text on phone: R U TXTN 2 MUCH IS IT REKIN UR SPELLIN??

This guide will help you to:

■ Learn and remember the correct way to spell the mistakes teachers highlight on your work.
■ Find the spelling strategies that suit your learning style.
■ Identify your target areas.
■ Know what to do if you can't spell a word.

There is a lot of space in this booklet for you to add your own words.

Have a go at all the techniques until you find the right ones for you.

1. Syllables

➜ Break the word into syllables.
➜ Say the word and count the syllables.
➜ Write the word. Draw a line between each syllable.
➜ Make sure that you can spell each syllable.
➜ Say and write the whole word.

2. Tackle the Tricky Bit

➜ Look carefully at the word.
➜ Underline the tricky bit.
➜ You know the rest, so just learn the tricky part.
➜ Say and write the whole word.

3. Use Your Spelling Knowhow

You know how to spell hundreds of words. If you can't remember how to spell something try to make a connection between the word and a word you do know how to spell.
Use your knowledge of rhyme, rules and patterns.

➜ Say the word. Find a word that you can spell that sounds similar.
➜ Write down the word that sounds similar.
➜ Add or change letters until it looks like the word you want to spell.
➜ Say and write the whole word.

Figure 2.9 (ii) (iii)

4. Mnemonics

This word means a memory help. It works by getting your whole brain involved in remembering something.

➜ Think of a catchy way to remember the spelling.

➜ Here are some examples:

There is a rat in separate.
Necessary = 1 collar and 2 cuffs.
Because = Big Elephants Can Always Use Small Exits.

Warning! Sometimes people spend a lot of time coming up with extremely complicated mnemonics that they then forget!

5. The Old Favourite

LOOK

SAY

COVER

WRITE

CHECK

Figure 2.9 (iv) (v) Booklet

Handwriting

We live in an age where rightly or wrongly we are judged initially by our appearance and what we say. This extends to handwriting, which is in essence an extension of ourselves and unique. A weak and illegible script provides evidence to parents, teachers, peers, employers and the pupil that there is a problem, and can in some instances give a wrong impression of a pupil's innate ability. No pupil wants to have their written work regarded as immature, with this immaturity being reflective of their emerging adolescent self-image. Dyslexic learners can find the actual task of writing difficult. This is for a variety of reasons, including problems with gross and/or fine motor control, poor writing style and a difficulty with the formation and orientation of letters. Weak spelling can exacerbate the problem. If work is illegible then spelling errors cannot be identified and corrected. Even in this age of technology and word processing, correct letter production is important in the secondary school. Legible handwriting matters for examinations, confidence and self-image.

Handwriting is relatively easy to ameliorate by non-specialist teaching at home or at school or both. Targets can be clearly set that are SMART – that is, they are Specific, Measurable, Achievable, Realistic and Time-related.

Stages of assessment and target setting

- If a pupil has a handwriting problem that makes legibility difficult and is a cause for concern, the first step is for the responsible adult to assure the pupil that they are looking for handwriting improvement and not change. Some pupils panic when they think they will have to change their handwriting script drastically.

- After assuring the pupil that you are not going to force them into writing reams of letters, the next stage is to ask the pupil to go away and produce three copies or samples of handwriting. One sample is an example of best writing; the second is an example of everyday writing (the bread and butter writing); the third sample is a piece of writing written in a hurry.

- At this stage a note is made about the handedness of the pupil (right, left or ambidextrous).

The P stage

We call this the P stage because this is the Preliminary or Pre-writing part of the assessment. The pupil is observed before putting pen to paper for Posture, Pen and Paper.

Posture

Teachers and assessors need to look at how the pupil sits at the table or desk to write. Is he or she slouched over the table with one hand supporting the chin, or is he or she sitting in a relaxed but controlled manner? Are the feet firmly on the ground and is the chair at a good height in relation to the desk? Does the pupil look comfortable and not crunched up?

Pen grip

Note needs to be taken of the manner in which the pupil is holding the writing implement. There is a preferred grip for right handers (about two centimetres from the pen point) and another for left handers (about three centimetres from the pen point). Show pupils Figure 2.11 to illustrate where their fingers should be, and demonstrate yourself.

Ensure that the grip is relaxed and if necessary do exercises relaxing and then tightening up a grip so that the pupil can feel the difference as well as see it. Finally, a word is needed about the hooked left handed grip. If this is present by the time of secondary education, it is firmly established and hard to change. One way of encouraging the pupil to write in a less unorthodox and cumbersome manner is to give them a sloping board on which to practise, or let them use the

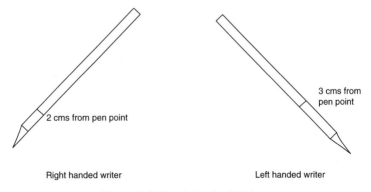

Right handed writer   Left handed writer

Figure 2.11 Handgrips for Writing

classroom white board. Writing with a hooked grip on an upright slope is difficult and this tactic might encourage a break in this habit.

Paper position

This refers to the position of the paper or writing book on the desk. Again there is a preferred position or slant of the paper in relation to the handedness of the writer. Right handers should slant their paper or book slightly to the left and left handers slightly to the right. At this stage it is important to point out to pupils that their non-writing hand is there to act as a balance, to give more control and act as an anchor. It is not there to prop up chins!

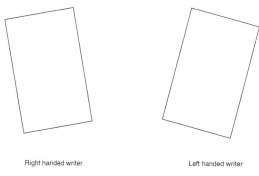

Right handed writer　　　　　Left handed writer

Figure 2.12 Paper Position

The E stage

We call this the E stage because we feel these elements play an Essential part in any programme for improving handwriting.

Cursive script

Whatever pupils, teachers or parents call it – joined up writing, cursive, real writing – the effect is the same. Cursive writing is more desirable for the emergent adolescent because it is mature, faster than printing, neater, usually more legible and age appropriate. Many pupils arrive in Year 7 of the secondary school with an immature printing script. There may be a variety of reasons for this, such as motor difficulties. However, there are some pupils who simply prefer to print. They have been taught how to write cursively but believe that their writing is neater and faster when printed. Printing has become a long-established habit. How do we convince these pupils that their writing will eventually be faster, more legible and more grown up if they persevere with the cursive script? How do we motivate them to try when it is obvious that they are not motivated, but they are getting increasingly unhappy with the status quo? One way we have found is to target cursive writing for them, pinpointing it for a short period of time and making the target very specific, e.g. 'You will write in joined writing for all lessons for the next two weeks and bring me examples of your written work in English, history and science as evidence you have done this. Date to be in by, 8 May.'

Pupils are likely to try this target even when they believe it will not make any difference to them in the long run. This is because it is only for a short time and it makes all the pertinent people in their life happy. It is a good idea to take a sample of the printed work before and after so that a comparison can be made. The pupil should see the improvement using cursive handwriting and note how their more mature hand is perceived by adults and peers. No teenager wants the script of a seven-year-old, however reluctant they are to make this change!

Dotting i's and crossing t's

This might seem like a target that does not matter on first glance, but we have included this in our E section, as we feel that it is essential to legibility. For example, the word 'taler', found in a piece of written work, was actually meant to be 'later'. The 'l' had been crossed instead of the 't' in a haphazard fashion. While this was not intentional, the effect was that it appeared as a spelling error and contributed to a loss of meaning.

Writing on the line

On first consideration this seems a very obvious target, but there are many pupils who struggle with keeping their writing on the line. With work on this simple target the improvement to written work can be substantial. The target appeals to pupils because it achieves maximum results from minimal effort, and they are not overwhelmed. It is cross-curricular and easy to remember to do, and provides success in a short period of time.

The S stage

We call this the S stage because it is more Specific. It includes detailed work on four main areas that can be chosen as appropriate to the individual difficulty:

- The *slope* or *slant* of letters.

- The *size* of letters in relation to each other.

- The *space* between letters and words.

- The *shape* of the letter and orientation.

The slope or slant of letters

This target is visually easy to illustrate to the pupil. It gives pupils choice over their style of writing. Pupils are asked to look at three options for the slope or slant of letters:

- All letters sloping upright: | | | | |

- All letters sloping to the right: / / / / /

- All letters sloping to the left: \ \ \ \ \

Pupils are asked to choose which of the above slants they want to adopt for their writing. They are told they cannot have a combination of all three.

The size of letters in relation to each other

This target, in our experience, is the one that takes the longest time to achieve and master. Pupils need to be given plenty of practice in writing letters that are relative in size to each other. Ascenders and descenders should initially be clearly accentuated. Small letters should be roughly half the size of the ascenders and descenders and be of a uniform size. We recommend using the commercial writing paper that has red lines and small blue middle lines. There is a tactile version of this available, which is suitable for multisensory learning.

The space between letters and words

The space between words should roughly be the width of the little finger or the size of a rounded letter such as 'o'. Bad spacing can lead to complete breakdown of legibility:

Th efir stda yofsp ringis thed aywhe nlam bsfro licin thef ields.

This is easily read when spaced properly.

The first day of spring is the day when lambs frolic in the fields.

Give the pupil some examples showing why it is important to space words correctly. Get pupils to make up their own sentences and then space them both correctly and incorrectly. A game can be devised based on this skill.

The shape of letters and orientation

The targets we set in this area are straightforward and direct.

- All closed letters should be closed, such as a, o, d, p, g, b.

- All open letters should be open, such as u, y, v, c, w, m, n.

- All small letters start at the top.

- Teach either b or d, but not together. Make sure that any teaching is multisensory.

Whole-school policy on handwriting

Most schools have a whole-school policy on spelling and there should also be one on handwriting. The aim of any handwriting policy is to provide a consistent whole-school approach to written work that gives pupils clear expectations, reduces anxiety and raises the standard of handwriting and presentation across the curriculum. A few teaching objectives successfully completed are better than more ambitious plans that cannot be fulfilled. There is always a danger of being over-prescriptive. Handwriting policies should be based on the four main themes of:

- legibility;

- speed;

- endurance;

- quality.

Presentation should be standardised across the curriculum, with clear expectations agreed and drawn up about the use of a ruler to underline headings, labelling of diagrams and the use of space on the page.

Postscript

If a dyslexic pupil is having significant problems with legibility and handwriting, then clearly written work should be accepted when submitted in a word-processed form. At university or college all work has to be submitted word-processed. The dyslexic pupil can also sit GCSE examinations using a word processor if appropriate, and special arrangements should be applied for, with permission granted by the relevant examination board. The school must ensure, and provide evidence, that the pupil has used word processing as an acceptable alternative to written work for a period of time and is practised in so doing.

Chapter 3

Dyslexia and English Grammar

Grammar is concerned with words and their usage. Just as a carpenter needs tools to make furniture, nails and glue are also required to hold the pieces of furniture together. Words are the bricks of our language; grammar is the mortar that binds them together. Dyslexic pupils need to be taught English grammar in a structured, explicit and multisensory way. The logic that runs through the backbone of grammar provides a blueprint for teaching. Letters lead to words, words lead to sentences, sentences lead to paragraphs and paragraphs lead to pages, articles, essays, reports and books. From this base, the interwoven threads that make up the umbrella term of 'grammar' radiate laterally. This is a perfect structure for the lateral thinker and dyslexic mind.

Word structure

Words are the tools of our language. We encourage pupils to take an active interest in words themselves. We do this through modules in etymology, discussing roots of words, prefixes, suffixes and compound words. Our dyslexic pupils enjoy playing with words and find this activity challenging and motivating. They are curious about words and find the experience of discovering, for instance, where words and their roots come from both fascinating and helpful. They can fit the information they discover into a cross-curricular context tying in with humanities, modern foreign languages, science, technology and mathematics. Pupils can be investigators and work

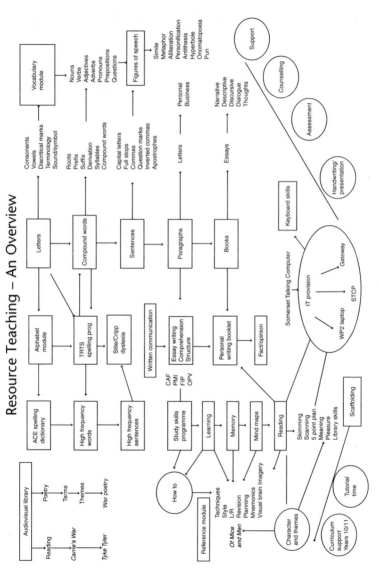

Figure 3.1 A Teaching Programme Overview

out patterns in words, looking at similarities, differences and common threads in spelling. Dyslexic pupils enjoy manipulating words. Prefixes and suffixes should be taught logically, systematically, explicitly and in a visual way whenever possible. Pupils can then use prefixes and suffixes to change the meaning and function of words in sentences with ease and confidence. When pupils experiment with words such as they do with these activities, they extend their vocabulary both orally and in a written sense. They not only become more confident with words themselves, but the additional familiarity they experience brings with it the bonus of self-esteem and success. No one wants to be restricted to saying and writing a simple code and denied access to the richness and variety of language that others use, because of fear of failure and a lack of confidence in handling language. We believe that the inclusion of language usage is as important as the inclusion of reading and membership of the reading club of life. A thorough grounding in word structure is therefore an essential component of any English grammar programme.

Punctuation

Without punctuation it is difficult to make sense of what is written. Punctuation is an aid to communication. Without it, the sense of what is to be conveyed through the written word can be lost and ambiguous. Some dyslexic pupils do not make the connection between punctuation used in speech and punctuation used in writing. They do not realise, unless it is explicitly pointed out to them, that when we articulate we use pause, intonation and stress to make sense of what we are saying, thus making meaning clearer for the listener. This concept is fundamental for applying written punctuation.

For example, many dyslexic learners can tell you, quite accurately, that sentences start with a capital letter and end with a full stop. However, they do not apply this in their writing. Why not? One reason could be that they know *what* to do and *how* to do it, but not *when* to. A result of this is a tendency to 'scatter' capital letters and full stops liberally in paragraphs, sometimes without any apparent logic, just so that the passage is 'punctuated' and they are fulfilling a requirement. You can only end a sentence with a full stop and start a new one with a capital letter if you 'know' what a sentence actually is, and the point is similar for paragraphs. For example, many dyslexic learners 'know' that a paragraph should be indented and will tell you that. However, they do not have a visual image of exactly what a paragraph looks like. We have found that drawing out the shape of a paragraph and showing on it diagrammatically the key points does get over this difficulty and gives the pupil a better understanding of exactly what a paragraph should look like.

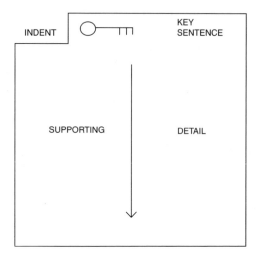

Figure 3.2 The Visual Paragraph

Other punctuation marks can be treated in a similar fashion. For instance, the visual difference between a comma and an apostrophe is in the position of the same mark on the page. Apostrophes hang up on the upper line; commas sit on the lower line.

• A comma lies on the line

• An apostrophe hangs from the top line

Figure 3.3 The Apostrophe and Comma

Pupils need much overlearning and explicit teaching if they are to use punctuation successfully, efficiently and effectively. Do not underestimate what needs to be taught. For example, 'A question mark is used at the end of a sentence that asks a question. Question marks do not need their own full stop as they have one included in their form.' This seems obvious perhaps, but is an example of how explicit you need to be when teaching punctuation. Remember, what is obvious to the English specialist will not be so obvious to the dyslexic pupil.

'Punctuation Detectives' is a game we play with Year 7 pupils when teaching this topic. Pupils are armed with punctuation marks, symbol/name correspondence and a code of punctuation marks, and are given their own punctuation mark to investigate. Pupils are encouraged to look in newspapers, magazines and books for examples of the punctuation mark they have been allocated. They make collections of how their mark is used, grouping together different aspects of their mark. The idea is to build a picture that can be turned into a mind web showing all aspects of their discovery.

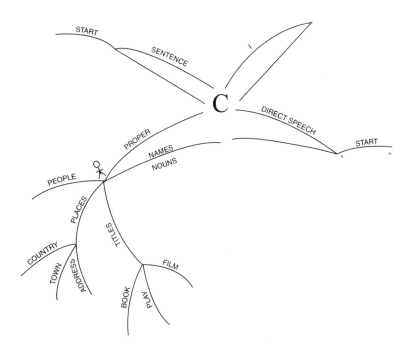

Figure 3.4 Capital Letters

Parts of speech

Nouns, verbs, adjectives, pronouns, adverbs, prepositions and conjunctions are the building blocks of our language. A thorough knowledge of parts of speech, with its terminology and usage, empowers pupils and provides the familiarity with language and its usage that is so important. Do not assume that dyslexic pupils 'know', for instance, what a noun is, or indeed how to use it. This must be taught explicitly, visually and in a structured way. A good grounding and teaching in basic grammar pays dividends. It can lead to an innate understanding of how words relate to each other, resulting in richness in both spoken and written language. Dyslexic pupils should be taught and know automatically that:

- nouns are naming words;

- verbs are doing words;

- adjectives are describing words;

- pronouns stand instead of the noun;

- adverbs add extra meaning to the verb;

- conjunctions are joining words;

- prepositions are placed in front of a noun usually to denote place or position.

These parts of speech can be taught effectively using colour coding and visual pegs on which to hang the concepts. Dyslexic pupils need to understand, for example, exactly what a verb is and the importance of it in the structure of a sentence. They may have problems learning 'parts of speech' in rote fashion because it involves name/symbol correspondence, which historically is an area of weakness in many dyslexic profiles. They therefore need to be taught 'parts of speech' in a multisensory, sequential and structured way.

Sentence structure

We recommend that any work on sentence structure is also built up systematically and runs alongside the module on parts of speech. Thus, work on conjunctions and the part they play in joining sentences together in written language would fit into simple sentence structures, developing further into compound and complex sentences. Working with verbs provides another opportunity for transference. The agreement of verb and subject would fit into all sentence structure work. This interrelationship and interdependence should be pointed out to all pupils, so that they do not regard individual modules in isolation. All transference of learning needs to be explicitly stated. Use as many technical and linguistic terms with the pupils as you wish. As long as the terms are fully explained in the way in which the pupil learns, and understood by him or her, there is no need to dilute or simplify. Differentiation can be used to ensure that inclusion is met.

Syllables

All pupils should be given a thorough grounding in syllables and syllable division. An understanding of the part syllables play in our language helps reading, spelling and the pronunciation of words. When we teach syllables initially, we use the analogy of a bar of chocolate, pre-formed into 'chunks', to establish exactly what a syllable is. This is a powerful multisensory image and one that pupils can readily absorb and retain, as it is visual and within the personal experience of most pupils. They are asked if they can put a large bar of chocolate into their mouths at once and enjoy it. Pupils usually comment that it would be difficult to get the entire chocolate bar in all at once, as the bar would hurt the inside of the mouth. It would therefore not be an easy task and not very enjoyable. However, if the same chocolate bar was broken down into the pre-formed chunks, the pupil could easily manage to eat the whole bar and enjoy it. This is a good analogy to use for breaking down words into syllables! Another useful tip for counting syllables in words is to speak the word clearly and at the same time tap the syllables out on a desk or table with the fingers. This enables the pupil to feel the syllable as well as hear the tap of the syllable. Always start counting with the same digit each time, so that it becomes automatic. We suggest the pupil uses the thumb. This means the pupil does not have to count the syllables until after the word has been broken down. (It is difficult to count and say the syllables at the same time.) Once the word has been broken down, then the fingers tapped can be counted, starting with the thumb; the number of syllables in the word can then be worked out.

Here is a suggested sequence for teaching syllables.

1. Listening to syllables in words.
2. CVC single syllable words (closed syllables).
3. CV words (open syllables).
4. Compound words (two single words joining).
5. Vowels and syllables : relationship.
6. Syllable division (closed syllables): CVVC.
7. Syllable division (open syllables): VCV.
8. VCE rule (e makes the vowel long).
9. Final syllables.
10. Suffixes and prefixes.

Plurals

When teaching plurals, which we consider essential, again the maxim is to teach in a systematic and explicit way, involving multisensory techniques whenever and wherever possible. Do not assume, for instance, that the pupils understand what is meant by the terms 'singular' and 'plural'. This needs to be spelt out as many of the so-called 'plural rules' rely on adding to or changing the singular form. It is therefore imperative that the fundamental principle of knowing the difference between singular and plural is firmly established at the beginning. Plural rules then need to be built up from this base, and taught in a logical fashion, with an emphasis on ascertaining the most likely plural from the singular form. Most dyslexic learners we have taught enjoy and very quickly and easily assimilate the plural rules. We give them plenty of practice in making plurals, collecting and matching them, as well as identifying plural rules in magazine articles, books etc. We have compiled a module on plurals, which systematically builds up the plural rules, with opportunities built in for overlearning. This culminates in a test, but a test with a difference, in that the pupils are given the question paper before the test. The pupils are given it as homework so that they can see the questions and learn what we want them to retain. They then sit the test knowing what they need to know to answer successfully. This technique has proved to be very popular, as pupils learn only what they know they need to achieve success. It appears to be motivational and the directed approach allows them to make efficient use of their memories. It also appeals to them because they feel they are somehow beating the system!

Figures of speech

Writers or speakers use figures of speech in order to make ideas more vivid, clear and forceful. Most figures of speech are based on the use of comparison, emphasis or contrast, and they need to be taught explicitly to dyslexic pupils to enrich their language and empower them. Dyslexic learners frequently have the ability to describe or use language in an unusual and powerful way, but they seem to need permission to do so. The insight into language frees them from the constraint of writing only what they can spell, as opposed to what they can think.

Figures based on comparison

Simile
In its simplest form a simile is a comparison made between persons or objects that differ in every way except for one or two points. The words 'like' or 'as' are used. This somewhat obvious point needs to be explicitly stated and illustrated. Pupils can be asked to look at similes in detail and highlight the words 'like' or 'as'. They can be given exercises to identify similes from a variety of phrases and can also be encouraged to collect similes and identify them in the writing and articles of others. For instance, pupils will need to know why 'Jane is like Jill' is a comparison and not a simile or metaphor. They should be given opportunities to identify similes and metaphors in pieces of work, given examples with which to play and sort into groups and then be encouraged to use metaphors and similes in their own writing.

Metaphor
A metaphor can be described as a similar comparison to a simile but without the words 'like' and 'as'. Essentially, a metaphor is transference. Nouns, adjectives, verbs and adverbs can express metaphors. For example:

- Juliet is the sun. (Noun)

- Life is but a walking shadow. (Adjective)

- She is bursting with pride. (Verb)

- He spoke hotly. (Adverb)

If there are two metaphors in a sentence, they should be clearly and closely linked and deal with the same idea. If this is not done the sentence can end up with a 'mixed metaphor'. Again this should be explicitly taught to the class, with plenty of opportunities given to practise the skill.

Allegory, fable and parable

All these are really extended similes or sustained metaphors. An allegory is a long, narrative metaphor, usually with a moral. Bunyan's *The Pilgrim's Progress*, recounting Christian's journey to the Holy Land (which in reality is man's life on earth), is a good example of an allegory. A fable is a narrative where birds, animals and insects represent human beings in their activities and point to a moral. Aesop's *Fables* are good to use to explain this. Finally, a parable is the term used for biblical stories in the New Testament that teach a lesson. Again this can have a cross-curricular relationship and can be taught using an investigative approach.

Personification

This is the making into a person of an inanimate object. That is, inanimate objects or abstract ideas are given the attributes of a person.

- Murder stalked through the village.

- Winter gripped the trees with icy hands.

Many dyslexic pupils have wonderful visual images in their heads that they can use in their writing when they are empowered with a working knowledge of figures of speech.

Apostrophe

This is a special kind of personification in which an object or idea is addressed as a living person, or may be addressed as if it was an absent or deceased person.

- O wild, west wind!

All pupils can benefit from being taught about these figures of speech and being encouraged to use them in their writing.

Figures based on emphasis by contrast or surprise

Antithesis

Antithesis is contrast. It frequently emphasises opposites. Use good strong examples to illustrate this figure of speech, such as:

- Youth is nimble, age is lame.

- More haste, less speed.

Epigram

An epigram is an inscription that often employs contrast. Most proverbs, for instance, are epigrams – that is, short witty remarks. The essence of an epigram is its brevity and unexpectedness. This appeals to many dyslexic learners, who may use this figure of speech with great skill.

- There is no fool like an old fool!

Hyperbole

Hyperbole is exaggeration. Exaggeration can be used successfully for particular effect and can be a powerful tool.

- He is as old as the hills.

Paradox

A paradox is an apparent contradiction of accepted facts and thus all the more striking by its truth. Many dyslexic learners we have taught enjoy the subtleties of using paradox.

- The child is father to the man.

- Our enemies are often our best friends.

Oxymoron

This is the contrast of sharp exact opposites united in the same phrase and so is more compressed and sharper than a paradox. Many dyslexic learners find oxymorons fascinating and humorous. Here are some examples that have caught their eye. They are well worth teaching.

- Great Britain.

- A silent scream.

- Sweet sorrow.

- Pretty ugly.

- Amicable divorce.

- Bad luck.

- Civilised warfare.

- Definitely maybe.

- Future history.

- Fighting for peace.

- Ill health.

- Long shorts.

Figures based on the appeal or effect of sound

Alliteration
This comes from 'litera', meaning 'letter', and is the use of the same letter to create an effect.

- 'S' has a hushing effect, as in 'to sit in solemn silence'.

- 'F' has a rustle sound, as in 'forest ferny floor'.

- 'W' has a whistling sound, as in 'whale's way' and 'wind like a whetted knife'.

- 'D' and 'T' are dentals with a heavy sound, as in 'down dropped the sails'.

- 'P' has popping sounds and 'B' explosive sounds.

Onomatopoeia

Onomatopoeic words sound similar to the subject they describe, as in 'the *buzz* of innumerable bees'. This is a favourite with dyslexic learners. They enjoy playing and experimenting with sounds and words.

Pun

This is a play on words that have more than one meaning. Examples are 'Is life worth living? That depends on the liver!' and 'A cannonball shot off his legs so he laid down his arms!'

Teaching and learning about figures of speech can be fun and in our experience is not a chore. They can be taught in a multisensory way with an emphasis on a 'hands on' approach, playing with and investigating words, idioms and phrases. Teaching grammar to all pupils equips them with the tools to handle their language.

Chapter 4

Creating a Dyslexia-friendly Learning Environment

When approaching the teaching of dyslexic pupils for the first time it is easy to think automatically about reading and spelling weaknesses. The jokes and misguided public perceptions have reduced dyslexia to a 'condition' that makes people into bad spellers and slow readers. It is important to realise that there are many more strengths and weaknesses to consider when setting out to ensure that dyslexic pupils have a positive experience in your classroom. We have a set of general principles that are the premise to any staff development work and that preface information booklets we give to staff. The teaching strategies are:

- Dictation should not be used.

- Copying from the whiteboard will be difficult for pupils; it may also be inaccurate.

- Whenever possible give handouts and allow pupils to highlight them.

- When correcting spelling errors be sympathetic. Do not draw attention to every one. Tackle the most common errors first, and those you have been teaching.

- Split errors up into syllables in order to reinforce the pupil's awareness of them. This is specifically referred to in statements.

- Long-term projects should be broken down into chunks where necessary.

- Give praise for effort as well as attainment.

- Do not ask pupils to read aloud unless they volunteer to do so.

- Help should be given in an unobtrusive way.

- New concepts should be explained, reinforced and overlearned.

- Aim for short achievable tasks with in-built success, to boost self-image.

- Record homework in planners if asked or if you feel there is a need.

- Check understanding of instructions by keeping them brief and asking pupils to repeat them.

- Use the 'buddy' system for instructions if pupils have a problem with them. Pupils must repeat instructions to their partners before starting the work.

- Allow pupils time to talk through their ideas before starting any lengthy written task.

- Use peer or sixth form support.

- Insist that pupils place their hands on their desks, face the front and maintain eye contact when you are giving instructions.

- Insist that pupils write the date in full, 'classwork' and a title on the top of each piece of work.

This may seem like a daunting list of 'you must not . . . '. However, we have many examples of good practice that offer staff alternative ways of working and, as we have previously stated, what helps dyslexic pupils also helps other learners.

Oracy

Using oral tasks as part of the planning, writing and drafting process is crucial in any English class. It instils confidence, generates and legitimises ideas and ensures that pupils with verbal strengths but who have literacy difficulties have opportunities to achieve. It has to be a fixed part of a teaching repertoire that is used in a consistent way. Pupils need to know that it will be part of the process and they need to be shown how to use the time effectively.

The English teacher needs first to ensure that ground rules have been established. The atmosphere has to be one of trust and mutual respect. When meeting a new group for the first time it is important that the teacher gets to know them and that they know the teacher before any oral work that involves risk taking is attempted. When a suitable atmosphere has been established, oral tasks become invaluable. Pupils benefit from reading work out in whole class or small group situations. Hearing paragraphs, full stops and commas as they occur naturally can teach pupils how to use punctuation. We have found that when a group works well together, the advice and support they offer each other really makes an impact. They are all in similar places on a continuum and they naturally offer small steps that may not have occurred to an English teacher who is at a completely different level. As they are members of a peer group they are often the correct audience for pieces of work. If this is the audience to which they want their short story to appeal, then the opinion of this audience is much more important to them than that of the teacher.

Using oral work as preparation for analytical, persuasive or informative written tasks helps for a number of reasons. The most important reason is that it gives thinking time to those who need it and therefore prevents panic. All pupils are able to gain confidence from the knowledge that they have ideas to use. Sharing ideas is a great leveller. Some dyslexic pupils find starting work quickly extremely difficult. They have the experience of getting things wrong in the past fixed in their minds. If they have heard what other people think or are going to do, then they have confirmation that their own approach to the task is correct. Their work is often more successful if they have been allowed to discuss their ideas in informal or formal situations. Pupils are willing to invest time and energy in planning a task because they are talking; usually this doesn't have negative connotations for them. When the whole class plans the work, they will own it.

In English, exploration of character, plot, theme and atmosphere are often essential skills. Drama activities can develop empathy and a deep moral understanding of a piece of literature. Tasks are numerous and can lend themselves to any text. Less confident pupils gain from watching others or having an instrumental role in the planning of a piece.

Planning

Teaching pupils how to plan and to choose the style of planning that suits them ensures that they can start writing in class or in examination situations. The habit of planning in a practised and familiar way reduces panic and enables pupils to use paragraphs more effectively. Teach very simple planning techniques. These techniques have to be taught from the start and used consistently in order to reinforce this skill as a basis of good writing.

In English, pupils have to demonstrate their ability to write in five different styles: descriptive, imaginative, persuasive, informative and analytical. They also have to show that they are able to choose and use a number of formats appropriately. The main formats required are reports, speeches, formal letters, articles, leaflets, poetry, advertisements and scripts. If you build confidence in their ability to recognise and employ these formats it will make them better writers. Ensuring that they know the range of the repertoire required of them also makes it less daunting.

Pupils are taught to plan their descriptive writing by using their senses as the first parts of the branches of a mind map. They start with what they can see, hear, smell, taste, touch and feel. They are taught that touch and feel are very different. It is explained that some branches won't be appropriate in every case but they should always put them down on the mind map to help them to remember the six categories. The order of the branches translates naturally into the order of their paragraphs. They can start superficially with what they can see and then develop their ideas until they write at a deeper level about what their feelings are.

The planning of imaginative writing starts in a similarly simple way. They use four of the question words as their first branches:

- The **who** branch develops into their ideas about characters. They are taught that they should have no more than four for a short story. These include hero, villain and victim. They are encouraged to gain an insight into the characters' personalities. To support this process, they are asked to write down five powerful adjectives about each character.

- The **what** branch develops the beginning, middle and end of the story. It is possible to develop their understanding of the principles behind all stories by teaching them to think in terms of harmony, problem and resolution. They are taught to plan using the following prompts as substitutes for beginning, middle and end as they become more sophisticated planners: calm–storm–calm; peace–conflict–peace; harmony–villain–harmony; happiness–problem–happiness; normal life–event–normal life.

- The **when** branch is a reminder that a short time frame needs to be selected, as this is critical when writing a short story. This branch is also used to reinforce the choice of tenses when writing. The tense in which they are going to write has to be specified at this stage in their planning. If they find this problematic the plan can be used to open dialogue about their choice.

- The **where** branch is used to prompt them to choose a maximum of three locations and to write down five powerful adjectives about each place.

This method may seem over-prescriptive. It is used to scaffold pupils who struggle to start writing, and as a springboard to ensure that every pupil starts writing. The narrow focus is also important in assisting dyslexic pupils to organise their ideas. Ensuring that they know about cliffhangers and other ways to break conventional narrative patterns is also important as they develop their confidence as writers. Some dyslexic pupils can only gain this confidence if they have been taught ways to start writing and therefore achieve success for their efforts. It is also essential to ensure that pupils know that plans and patterns are scaffolds that can be jettisoned as they develop their skills.

The ability to write in the three remaining styles – informative, persuasive and analytical – can be broken down into a number of skills that need to be explicitly taught.

- Pieces required to demonstrate the ability to persuade, inform or show understanding need to start with ideas. This is an ideal time to use oral work to ensure that pupils have access to a number of ideas.

- Mind-mapping skills may have been established in previous school years. Pupils need to be reminded how to use this technique to organise and develop their ideas. Model this skill by using Mind maps© on the whiteboard or on flip charts. Use colour, symbols and drawings.

- The next step needs to be the organisation of these ideas into a logical sequence. Introduction, develop, develop, develop and conclusion can provide a good starting point. This is a five-paragraph structure for letters, reports, essays etc.

- Then pupils have to be taught formats. These formats should be revisited as often as possible. Examples from pupils who write well are good tools to reinforce correct layouts. These can be laminated, used as a wall display or bound as a book of examples. This gives an added incentive, as it shows how the teacher values and celebrates good work. It makes the ability to write correctly in each genre feel attainable.

- These pieces of work are most successful when pupils are given a specific scaffold or writing frame to work through. We use the word scaffold to mean a worksheet or whiteboard guidance that provides paragraph starters and guides pupils through a piece of work. These are especially important when pupils write essays. The word 'essay' strikes terror into the heart of many pupils. They are familiar with and often enjoy writing narrative, but the tone, format and vocabulary required when writing essays can be daunting.

Drafting

Drafting has to be taught as an explicit skill. Pupils will often think that rewriting is all that is required when they are asked to redraft their work. This can even be quite a stressful and emotional time for pupils who have struggled to complete the task set.

Redrafting work has to have a context and a clear focus. Whatever the level of difficulty experienced by the pupil, they need to be given one or two SMART targets in order to see the purpose of redrafting. It is important that the work itself has a clear, explicit purpose. If pupils are demonstrating that they have learnt how to write in paragraphs and their work shows that they have succeeded in doing this, then they deserve praise. It is extremely tempting to use all written pieces as a reason to work at a spelling pattern or rule or as a reason to assess handwriting targets. Addressing and helping to ameliorate these two common problems caused by dyslexia is important. Teachers must make it part of their marking strategy to disregard them when other English skills are being assessed. Pupils will become demoralised very quickly if they feel that everything they do in English is secondary to the problems caused by dyslexia. The importance of good planning and scaffolds is reinforced when discussing redrafting. Teachers can revisit the plan with the pupil in order to support their constructive criticisms. Peer assessment is also strengthened if pupils have something to refer to with language that lends itself to practical support. For example, the imaginative writing plan prompts pupils to think about powerful adjectives, tense agreement, organisation and development of plot and the number and type of characters. This provides a framework that can be used to structure assessment and set SMART targets.

We have found the idea of teaching pupils the difference between editors and authors in the realm of published works extremely helpful when teaching redrafting. We teach pupils that published work means work for public consumption, and it is therefore special and different from work for their files or exercise books. We publish our pupils' work in a number of ways: on wall displays throughout the school and in our classrooms; in books that have been bound together; by laminating work; and by posting work on the school's website. Our pupils know that this work has to be edited to a different level from their usual work. This work is usually word-processed, which ensures that their patience with redrafting is prolonged. As authors of the work they improve it by using targets suggested by the teacher or their peer group. They also use the spelling and grammar checkers on their computers. They then employ the skills of an editor to help them to achieve work that is of a high enough standard to be published. Editors in our situation are other pupils, the teacher, sixth form in-class support or teaching assistants. Editors only change spelling, punctuation and grammar (SPAG); they do not alter the content of the work. We have found that this works because it legitimises intervention and ensures that pupils don't lose their sense of ownership of their work. We have found that drawing parallels with Roald Dahl, of whom they have all heard, helps a great deal. As part of our Year 7 initial unit of work on autobiographies and biographies we show a documentary about him in order to motivate them. The documentary details his literacy difficulties and his reliance on his editor to correct his spelling and punctuation. Pupils have a concrete example of an extremely successful author who used the process we are advocating. It is important that all pupils' work is edited before it is printed. Even pupils who have very few literacy difficulties must have their work checked if all pupils are going to believe in this way of working. It can be time consuming but it is only for published work, which need not be generated more than twice a year from any one class.

Presentation of work

As with all methods that help and support dyslexic pupils, the teacher's attitude to presentation has to be explicitly taught and consistently reinforced. Presentation of work is not just handwriting. As previously explained, there are certain weaknesses that have to be addressed. If the teacher has set targets and is addressing handwriting problems assessment of handwriting can be disregarded. This is an area where we have found that the establishment and reinforcement of high expectations are crucial.

All pupils benefit from being taught and reminded to follow certain rules regarding presentation. For example, all headings should be underlined using a ruler. Basic presentation standards may seem so obvious that the teacher doesn't feel the need to make them explicit. However, good practice in presentation is only obvious when you have good literacy skills. If a pupil revises from their exercise book they quickly learn how to make things clear by setting them out in a certain way. Pupils learn that diagrams should be labelled in a set way and that titles and dates are essential. If pupils don't or can't revise from their notes then they are in a vicious circle.

Organisational problems will also have an impact on dyslexic pupils' presentation of their work. Experience has shown that dyslexic pupils often lose or forget equipment. Some ensure that they have their exercise book for each lesson with them by keeping them in their bags at all times – even when their football boots are in there too! It is important to remove obstacles caused by dyslexia and we have found some simple things that have helped:

- We always circulate a red pen and ruler around the class at the beginning of each piece of work. It is a physical prompt that reminds pupils about the rule. It also prevents the disruption caused by a discussion about why pupils don't possess their own equipment.

- We keep pupils' exercise books in class unless they are set homework.

- We supply pupils with plastic book covers to protect their exercise books.

These three simple steps have helped.

We have found that outlining good practice and demanding that pupils follow our guidelines generates success. When pupils see that their work can improve even if they are still unhappy with their handwriting, it is encouraging and motivating.

While maintaining high expectations of presentation, pupils also have to be taught that literacy is an adaptable tool. As previously stated, they need to be explicitly taught that there are a multitude of purposes for reading and writing. The context of the task has an impact on the level of skill involved. We have found that many dyslexic pupils think that their spelling must always be accurate and their handwriting must always be neat. This stilts their planning work and slows them down when note taking. Pupils should be encouraged to label their work clearly with its purpose, enabling other staff and parents to see that the level of presentation is legitimate. Alternative ways of presenting notes in exercise books should be offered, such as Mind maps©, bullet points or pictures.

The classroom

Workspaces can become dyslexia-friendly very easily. We offer advice about organising workspaces at home to pupils and parents and we therefore have to model this organisation in our own classrooms. We use clear labels that help pupils to remember where to put things, and ensure that there is time at the beginning and the end of each lesson for pupils to store or retrieve equipment and books. Labelling learning aids and allowing easy access to them can also prevent stigma and embarrassment. We ensure that *ACE Spelling Dictionaries*, Irlen's filters and spelling tablemats are available without request.

We have found that wall displays can be used to reinforce learning. Word walls, which are spelling banks displayed on classroom walls, have become popular recently. These are useful aids if they are clear and visible. Printing them on a background colour other than white will cut down glare and will help pupils with Irlen's syndrome. Pupils should also have tablemats available because of visual memory problems.

The majority of our wall displays are celebrations of final, published work. We ensure that they are perfect in order to prevent criticisms from other pupils and staff about poor spelling. However, we also ensure that there is a constantly changing section of wall that shows 'Work in Progress'. This section shows Mind maps© and texts that are being annotated to aid understanding and recall. We believe that this section is important because it models the learning process across year groups and ability ranges and it legitimises techniques with which pupils are unfamiliar. We also feel that it reinforces the idea of the use of literacy as an adaptable tool. The space to experiment and brainstorm in their exercise books is echoed on the classroom walls.

In our school the 'published' work of our pupils is also displayed in many of the 'public' areas, such as the library, corridors and ICT rooms. This raises their profile and illustrates their capabilities, given the right guidance and support, to staff.

Some of the ideas we have stated here may seem obvious. We will be extremely pleased if they do to you and if you carry out this good practice already. We have seen this methodology work. The idea of teaching pupils with this complex learning difficulty can be daunting. We have found that a teacher's willingness to make minor changes to their approach to teaching English can make a great deal of difference to dyslexic pupils and have a positive effect on all pupils.

Chapter 5

Developing English Skills for GCSE

This chapter begins by establishing basic principles that are necessary to underpin all teaching at Key Stage 4 and then goes into specific ideas that will help when teaching Shakespeare, poetry or media.

Dyslexic pupils often find their English language and, to a lesser degree, their English literature examinations among the most difficult to pass. They can be allowed to see these subjects as the ones that examine their areas of weakness most critically. However, many dyslexic pupils enjoy and gain success in these subject areas. There are key aspects of teaching methodology that have ensured this progress.

A crucial first step in learning how to teach dyslexic pupils at Key Stage 4 is adjusting your mind set. Remember that English is a set of special codes with hundreds of rules. When we approach GCSE we try to get pupils to access the next set of codes on the continuum. We want to teach pupils what a sonnet is or how to analyse Shakespeare's language and stagecraft. Dyslexic pupils will want and be able to tackle these new concepts, but simultaneously they have to cope with their own particular dyslexic difficulties. As with every other subject area, in order to ensure successful access to our curriculum we have to alleviate dyslexic difficulties, not compound them. Just because we are teaching English, it doesn't mean that we have to abandon what our subject has to offer in order to focus on reading and spelling. When pupils get to this stage in their school career they need more than this in order to keep them interested in English. Our job is threefold: to encourage the continued development and practice of good coping strategies; to remove obstacles that prevent access to our subject; and, most importantly, to motivate and generate a willingness to analyse, study, read and write in English lessons.

At GCSE we are asking pupils to use and learn new vocabulary that has to be explicitly taught. This offers an opportunity to remind pupils of coping strategies for spelling. The difficulty of unfamiliar language provides a chance to remind pupils about syllables, mnemonics, memory aids and spelling rules. Colleagues have asked us if they can introduce words such as onomatopoeia, innuendo and oxymoron. We encourage this because pupils are entitled to learn about these techniques. Each subject area has its own key words and finds ways to allow pupils to use them. Topics such as photosynthesis cannot be dropped from the Key Stage 4 syllabus because thay are hard to spell. When these words are taught in a supported way, pupils feel empowered. In order to scaffold the learning of these words we take some practical steps. We use key word displays and laminated tablemats that link to the topic being studied. These can be added to with permanent overhead transparency pens. Blank laminated sheets can be used to create new mats. This makes pupils feel that the mats are relevant to them and to others.

Some of the tablemats have poetry words, discursive words, Shakespeare's techniques, *Stone Cold* words, powerful adjectives and media words. A similar technique that pupils like is the use of the free postcards that are available in cinemas, on which they write their own key words for a topic. Both of these techniques work better than word walls because the words are on the desk in front of the pupil. They can copy words letter by letter if necessary. Reading and retaining a whole word in their visual memories can be problematic for dyslexic pupils. This is why copying huge amounts from the whiteboard can be so difficult.

Time is another key factor. Build specific 'learning time' into your lessons. All pupils will benefit from the opportunity to learn how to spell and how to use these new terms. Refer to key ways to tackle spellings and allow pupils time to use their preferred coping strategies to learn a selection of words. Ensure that you give pupils time to investigate and make links between words.

The organisation of notes at GCSE poses huge problems for many dyslexic pupils. Pupils need to be reminded how to use colour coding, pictures, spider diagrams, mnemonics etc. They then need to be encouraged to experiment with these techniques and to jettison the ones that do not suit their learning style. We insist that pupils create a title page in their exercise books for every new novel or topic studied. This page should have a strong visual image that they can then associate with the topic. This can be a drawing, cut-outs or patterns. If we are working through a text we start by creating a contents page – for example, key words, storyline in brief, key events, characters, key quotes, themes, locations, techniques and evaluation. Each exercise book page is given a heading. This ensures that key notes are together at the start of the section and not punctuated by tasks or homework. Encourage pupils to use highlighters, colour, symbols and illustrations to give them ownership of this section. However, it may be necessary to supplement these notes with handouts if pupils find it difficult to read their own work. The purpose of making these notes is not the notes in themselves; it is the creation of a useful reference point for future revision or as the starting point for a piece of writing. We mark these notes carefully. Pupils will not want to revise from notes that are covered in red pen. Presentation is our main concern. We correct spelling if it is important to the learning. We correct the names of characters if we feel that the incorrect spelling will confuse the pupil when they study from the notes or if we feel that the examiner won't know whom they are talking about.

Another skill that has to be explicitly taught at the beginning of Year 10 is how to annotate texts. In English this is the first time they have really been asked to do this. The Welsh Joint Education Committee (WJEC) examinations that our pupils study are open book, and annotations are allowed to a certain extent. We have picked up a useful mnemonic that aids our teaching of annotation: COW (Comment On Words). Pupils tend to underline whole passages if we say that they are important, but using COW as a principle we have guided pupils into more useful underlining. Annotation is also aided if we use right brain skills. Symbols for key themes or characters are a useful shorthand and often appeal to dyslexic pupils. However, as with mnemonics, it is important to ensure that the symbols are not complicated and are applied consistently in order to prevent confusion and time wasting.

Planning and drafting skills must be explicitly taught to GCSE pupils. The provision of a scaffold is essential for pieces of coursework, but pupils must be taught how to produce their own scaffolds. Modelling good practice is a useful exercise. We use successful pieces of coursework from previous years for different texts. The class can use this model to produce a group scaffold for their own text. An extremely helpful task is also to look at examination-style questions and plan answers for homework on a regular basis. Sharing these plans reinforces the skill for those who are successful, but also provides extra modelling for those who are still developing their ability to plan.

Finding quotations that reinforce certain points is another crucial part of the planning process. We have found that this can be an extremely daunting task and, therefore when preparing coursework, group 'searches' can eliminate a great deal of stress. We make sure that pupils look for a number of alternatives for each point and encourage debate about who has the stronger quotation. We have found that this helps pupils to develop an interest in dissecting literature and also fosters the idea that many alternative interpretations are valid in this subject area.

We work hard to ensure that pupils use drafting as a useful tool. This skill is developed from Year 7 and good principles are in place by Year 10. However, redrafting coursework can be an extremely difficult thing to approach when a pupil has invested a significant amount of time in a first draft. Pupils are aware that coursework is going towards their final mark and it can become a highly emotive aspect of the course. We are always open and honest about GCSE grades. We feel that, as long as we are guiding pupils towards a higher grade through suggestions for redrafting, there is no justification for 'hiding' their grade from them. When pupils are aware of the English language and literature marking criteria they gain a helpful stimulus for redrafting. By offering the criteria in more concrete and accessible terms it is possible to help pupils to look at their work and the work of their peers and set achievable and relevant targets for improvement.

Many of our pupils have bought and use their own laptops to help them in school. This can be disastrous, as can using computers in general if rules are not established from the outset. We insist that work is backed up on to diskette and that hard copies are printed out. We have also found that making sure that work is saved with a useful title is crucial. Many pupils forget the significance of file names, or call all English work 'English'. Poor memory and organisational skills need support in some unexpected areas at times. If you establish the ground rules and are consistent in reinforcing them, then you have offered support if the problem is caused by dyslexia.

The choice of literature for pupils to study is central to the dyslexic pupil's experience during the GCSE course. We have found a number of texts successful. *Stone Cold* and *Our Day Out* are our current choices. They work for a variety of obvious reasons. Pupils enjoy studying short, modern texts with characters that are of a similar age to them. These stories contain a great deal of action and are shocking in places. They can also be studied using audio and videotapes to reinforce understanding and enjoyment.

Studying Shakespeare

Something that surprises a number of practitioners is that Shakespeare has also always been a favourite section of the course. We have had a great deal of success when we have taught a number of his plays to our dyslexic pupils. We are currently using *Romeo and Juliet*. This works well because pupils are often familiar with the plot because of the success of the Baz Luhrmann film version. It is about people around their age defying adults. Pupils enjoy analysing the characters in modern terms, comparing them to classmates or media figures. The play contains ample material for this kind of comparison. Pupils whose aural channels are stronger than their visual channels enjoy Shakespeare's language. We have found that dyslexic pupils respond well when they are taught about its features, such as puns, metaphors, oxymoron and innuendo. They actively search for examples to add to their notes. The play contains so many memorable quotations that they remember them quite easily. The cleverness of Shakespeare's language appeals to many dyslexic pupils because it tests their higher order thinking skills.

Our *Romeo and Juliet* scheme of work reveals some of the techniques that have helped our dyslexic pupils. We use prior knowledge as a starting point for a study of the play. Find out what pupils already know about Shakespeare and about the play. Many of them may have studied it in drama or may know the film extremely well. We ensure that we allow pupils to share their prior knowledge in order to allow an equal starting point for all pupils. We have found that male and female impressions of and ideas about the play differ a great deal. The key scenes that they remember from the Baz

Luhrmann film are split on gender lines to a certain extent. Many of the boys talk about the guns and the violence and the girls talk about the ball scene and Leonardo DiCaprio. However, what they all remember is more interesting. If pupils have seen the film they all comment on the costumes, the music and the ending of the play. The costumes and the music are excellent reference points that can be used to reinforce learning. They are highly stylised and turn characters such as Lady Capulet and Mercutio into caricature. They can be used to access right brain skills in order to aid students' memories.

After establishing that pupils know a great deal about the plot, the characters and the themes of the play, we have to justify our reasons for studying the actual text. What extra things will they gain from this exploration of it? We then show pupils marking criteria rewritten in a pupil-friendly way. We discuss terms such as 'stagecraft' and start to build up vocabulary banks on tablemats. We have found that at this stage it is important to strike a balance between challenging pupils to want to analyse the play and ensuring that they are not put off by the prospect.

The next part of the scheme of work ensures that all pupils know the story. The prologue tells the whole story. We do the obvious thing and get the class to translate it into modern English. This translation is displayed in the classroom and is illustrated by one or two of the best artists after we have covered the scene to which the text refers. It is a useful reference point, especially when we return to the play to revise for examinations. It is important to explain why a Shakespearean audience needs the prologue. This is a useful introduction to the nature of the audience. We have found showing carefully selected extracts from *Shakespeare in Love* helpful. Pupils enjoy the idea that visiting the theatre, something they consider to be high culture, was once seen as a corrupting and dishonourable pastime. They have often been taught about Shakespearean theatres and life prior to Key Stage 4 but some of the more unwholesome and therefore intriguing aspects of the topic may have been omitted. There are many non-fiction books that can be used to support this part of the scheme. Our pupils get a feel for the period by reading about sanitation, medicine, crime and punishment, all topics that appeal to teenagers' thirst for unsavoury pieces of information!

After the introduction to the topic we cover the actual play in four weeks; that is, 12 lessons. We have found that keeping the time frame short is essential to maintain the interest of the students. We use prose summaries and film clips to move pupils from key event to key event. We use both Baz Luhrmann's and Franco Zeffirelli's versions of the play. Our pupils want to read the script aloud and this motivation is maintained if extracts are short and contain a lot of action. We allow pupils to practise before they read to the class. We try to keep the same pupils for the same characters, as this can be a useful memory aid. We have found that our initial choice of pupils has been crucial. However, there is a danger of excluding pupils if they are not good at reading aloud or if they are not selected. Ensure that these pupils are given 'starring' roles in other ways. We structure our oral tasks to enable this.

When planning our scheme we are aware that notes and tasks will be more helpful if they demand a variety of skills. We access the play through many channels: listening, reading, viewing, reasoning, prediction, empathy and physical tasks. This variety ensures that every pupil's preferred learning style will be catered for. Colour codes and symbols have helped us to look at the balance of tasks and we have readjusted tasks accordingly.

Our pupils study *Romeo and Juliet* for their WJEC examinations. They are required to write an essay for their language folios. We have found that their motivation is maintained if we complete this work after we have studied the whole play. The most successful essay subject we have used is a study of the stagecraft of Act 3, Scene 1, the fight scene. As this scene is a catalyst for so many subsequent events and is so full of action, pupils are able to write a great deal about character, language and the impact on the audience.

There are a number of texts that we have found useful to help us to teach *Romeo and Juliet*. Hodder & Stoughton has produced a graphic version of the play and an accompanying *Teachers' Guide to Romeo and Juliet*. We do not advocate the use of the graphic text with dyslexic pupils unless it is as a supplement. However, the *Teachers' Guide* has some useful worksheets that we have used to support our students. They are well illustrated and their text is clear and uncluttered. The suggested tasks appeal to a range of learning styles and help to clarify some difficult concepts. Our students are given Oxford versions of the play. This version is full of useful suggestions for activities and contains clear page-by-page modern prose summaries of the story.

Poetry

Poetry is an essential part of GCSE courses. Pupils have to produce poetry comparison essays and analyse unseen poetry in examinations. We have found a number of techniques useful when supporting pupils in this area. Pupils often find this part of the course extremely rewarding. Poetry is shorter than prose and dyslexic pupils can often remember key quotes and storylines quite easily, especially if the poems chosen make an impact because of their themes or language. Pupils are often intrigued if poets use language in new or unusual ways. Illustrating copies of poems with drawings, shapes or colours can be a useful starting point for discussions. We use structured oral sessions to mind map© ideas about **S**torylines, **T**hemes, **A**tmosphere, **T**echniques and personal **E**valuations. The mnemonic **STATE** is used to structure essays and is helpful in examinations. A class scaffold is produced. Pupils are given responsibility for finding key quotations to support ideas. Our pupils have enjoyed studying poems from a collection called *Parallel Poems*.

Media Studies

We teach media studies as a GCSE subject in its own right and as an aspect of the English course. We have tried to discuss study of the media in terms of its content on the English syllabus but sometimes we refer to the media studies course because we have learnt useful things when teaching dyslexic pupils in both situations.

Reading and analysing media texts is often an area that dyslexic pupils find difficult. We found that when we started to teach dyslexic pupils in a mainstream class situation they sometimes stood out as lacking key skills in this area. There can often be a gap between dyslexic pupils and their peers in their ability to decode written media texts. When they work in teams and use their aural skills the gap disappears. This is because the media rely on puns and other in-jokes that require very good reading and visual skills. When dyslexic pupils hear the joke they are often very quick to interpret and analyse it. Analysing television advertisements before looking at printed texts is useful for all pupils. They are often sophisticated and cynical analysts where TV ads are concerned because they have had such a lot of exposure to them. Newspaper articles can also be approached via television in order to highlight key concepts before tackling written texts.

In their written work our pupils are able to demonstrate clever and manipulative uses of language when supported. We have found that giving pupils time to talk through their ideas, and using video and audio equipment to allow them to record their ideas in ways other than writing, have given them the confidence to learn media skills. The lexicon of journalese appeals to them when they have had opportunities to explore it and play with language. We have found that using puns, emotive and sensationalist language and inventing quotations is appealing to all pupils when they can try out ideas on their peers in structured oral work. By the time our pupils are writing newspaper articles, advertisements and leaflets for examinations they are able to concentrate on the process of writing because the creative aspect of the task has been rehearsed and is clear in their minds.

We have found that teaching GCSE English and English literature to pupils who have dyslexia or other learning difficulties can be one of the most rewarding aspects of our work. It is our opportunity to develop their understanding and appreciation of the techniques and skills employed in our subject. It often enables us to see pupils enjoying reading key texts and writing in a range of styles. It can be the time when their confidence peaks and they feel successful. It can, however, also be a time of confusion, anxiety and stress. We start to demand that pupils demonstrate their understanding of even more complexities of the English language. We always try to remember that English is a 'code' that has been developed over many centuries. It is neither a natural nor an organic part of the world. Being good at something is often an accident of birth. As teachers or other good practitioners we are in on the 'code'. We know it really well and we legitimise it and demand that it is used by all. We must never assume that pupils are not intelligent or entitled to access to key parts of our culture because they haven't quite got to grips with the special 'code'. We have to alter our delivery in order to remove barriers to understanding, success and enjoyment.

Chapter 6

Preparing for and Succeeding with National Examinations in English

All pupils in England and Wales have to sit statutory examinations in English at 14 and again at 16. At 14 (Year 9) the Key Stage 3 statutory assessment tests (SATS) are reading and writing tests. At 16 (Year 11) the GCSE (General Certificate of Secondary Education) has separate papers in English language (reading, writing and comprehension) and literature.

English, especially the language paper, is perceived by dyslexic learners as one of the most difficult examinations to face in the secondary phase. This is because dyslexic pupils are being tested in an area where historically they have experienced the most difficulties and where areas of weakness lie. They are being tested on their weaknesses and not on their strengths. In addition, for many parents great value is put upon their offspring achieving a high grade or level in English. Employers and universities demand English as a prerequisite for entry to courses, jobs and opportunities. It is no wonder that against this background the term 'English' has so many emotional overtones and hang-ups for many dyslexic learners. Being tested on actual or perceived weaknesses lowers confidence levels and self-esteem dramatically.

All pupils are required to sit these exams in a written form. Many dyslexics are highly articulate and would be capable of passing the

English exam at a high grade if it was given orally. The problem for the English teacher is how to marry the able articulate dyslexic pupil with the written paper the external examiner will mark. Not only parents and employers but pupils themselves see success in English as a prerequisite and passport to doors of choice. For example it is required for entry to teaching, university, nursing and many other professions. Therefore parents, employers, interviewers and pupils put a lot of value on a good grade in English.

What can be done to help and support the dyslexic pupil to succeed in this crucial area? How can we help them to overcome the practical and emotional barriers that have been built up and seem at times insurmountable? Here is a story taken from Helen Rollason's autobiography *Life's Too Short*, which we use when pupils are stressed and anxious. We hope that it dispels dragons for them.

Are you sitting comfortably?

Once upon a time there was a young prince who, as princes so often do in stories like this, was wandering around distant lands looking for adventure. He came to a village which nestled at the entrance to a pass between two mountains. On top of one of these was a huge dragon breathing fire and smoke. The villagers were all weeping and wailing and the prince astutely discerned that all was not well with them. He asked what was the matter and they told him that their best fields and crops were through the pass in the next valley and that they couldn't reach them because it meant getting past the dragon. He asked them why nobody had tried to tackle the dragon. They replied that on three occasions they had nominated their best fighter for the task, but that the path up the mountain was so steep that in each case the man had fallen off and died before he reached the top.

The prince was not hugely courageous, but being a helpful prince, he offered to see what he could do. To start with he decided that the most important challenge was to make sure he didn't fall off the path. So he began to make his way up this very narrow path, removing loose stones and obstacles as he went. Every now and then he stopped and took some deep breaths to prevent himself panicking. He noticed that the scenery was quite beautiful up there. He carefully continued picking his way up the path enjoying the scenery as he went. To his surprise he suddenly found himself on the top of the mountain. He looked around and couldn't see the dragon anywhere. Plucking up his courage he called out, 'Come on, dragon, where are you?' and he heard a little squeak from close to the ground. Looking down, he saw that by his left foot was a tiny little animal which he picked up and found it was a baby dragon.

'Where's your big brother, little dragon?' said the prince. 'I've come up here to fight him.'

'There's only me here,' said the dragon.
'But you can't be the dragon that's frightening the whole village.'
'Oh yes, that's me.'
'Well how on earth can you do that?'
'I'm able to do it because of my name,' said the dragon.
'What is your name?'
And the dragon said, 'What Might Happen.'

From a distance, What Might Happen is terrifying and we get so frightened of it that we fall off the path before we ever meet it. However, if you live in the present and do what you can to the best of your ability, when you meet your dragons you will nearly always find that they are the ones that you can pick up and deal with.

We feel that stress has to be considered as a central issue in any discussion about dyslexia and English. As we have stated previously, there is a lot of emotional baggage associated with the term English and when this is linked to examinations the stress levels are compounded.

English + Exam = Double whammy of stress

Think about situations when you have felt stressed. Imagine going home late at night when there is not a soul about. How do you feel? Are you relaxed and confident that you can handle yourself? Do you feel threatened, vulnerable and on the alert for signs and sounds of danger? All your senses are alert and your body's chemical and physiological composition responds to the perceived situation. The reptilian brain is in full swing. These feelings are similar to those experienced by pupils in the classroom and examination room if they are feeling extreme stress and anxiety. No wonder they have problems in concentrating and focusing on what you want them to do and what they must do.

Confidence building cannot be a sticking plaster applied at the last minute. It should be proactively built into the English curriculum from the beginning of examination courses. We have found that working from the premise 'you can do this well' and then empowering pupils with the skills to deliver makes them not only feel good about themselves but enjoy what they are doing. Experiencing the richness of both language and literature in a positive, enthusiastic learning environment breeds confidence. Building foundations from what pupils are good at, such as oracy, and approaching their weaknesses through scaffolding techniques ensures a safety net of skills. This is the philosophy behind our English teaching and we put this into practice through a number of tried and tested methods. First, transparency is essential. Pupils need to know what exactly is required of them during the course. We always share the vital pieces of information with our pupils in order to give them ownership of and responsibility for their learning:

- A knowledge of the syllabus and where they are, where they have been and where they are going.

- Numerical information about the breakdown of examination papers and coursework.

- Explicit marking criteria supported by models of good practice and perhaps opportunities missed through poor planning and/or drafting.

- Coursework tasks that are compulsory for success and provide an opportunity to achieve outside the examination hall.

- How to move forward by learning about learning.

- Pupils should know what level or grade they are achieving at a point in time.

We believe that we should mark realistically right from the beginning. This is a controversial issue and one that runs the risk of damaging the confidence that we are so keen to foster. However, if handled sympathetically and constructively pupils respect and respond to an honest appraisal of their current functioning, in the belief that improvements are expected and will be supported. The idea that only higher grade passes are valid is not acceptable to us. We recognise that for some of our pupils a pass at grade D, E, F or G is a huge achievement. What is important is that we have high expectations for all our pupils, based on individual strengths and weaknesses.

For some pupils the actual physical aspects of the examination are a problem. They have to sit in a hall under timed and strictly supervised conditions. In addition, they have to handle and answer questions that are produced in an official and in some instances unfamiliar paper. We feel that it is very important that our dyslexic learners and, indeed, all pupils have plenty of practice and become familiar with handling examination papers and examination words.

This is another part of our English code that has to be explicitly taught. Examination words can be specific to exams and are not usually found in everyday conversation or even in the classroom. Pupils need to meet these words regularly so they know what is required of them and how to do it. Inclusion means not being excluded and part of the English teacher's job is to enable access to technical vocabulary. As teachers we recognise that examination words are part of this vocabulary.

Recognition that there is a repertoire of skills in English that will be examined is a positive and releasing experience for some pupils. These are the pupils who have built a mountain as high as Everest around English and who do not have a realistic appraisal of what is expected unless it is explained to them and they understand. For example, in paper one of the WJEC GCSE language examination they have to write four comprehension answers, a piece of description and a story. Armed with this knowledge, and given opportunities to practise beforehand, they are much better prepared psychologically and practically.

We help pupils by initially providing structures to underpin any weaknesses in time management and organisational skills. We are explicit about what we want them to do, when we want them to do it, how they can do it and why the work is valid and important for them and their ultimate success. This is the essence of good practice.

Preparation of planning

Just because a pupil is in your lesson do not assume that they will remember what has been taught unless you use a multisensory approach and build overlearning and reinforcement into your teaching syllabus. It may need to be taught in a different way, recognising the different learning styles in the classroom.

There is provision built into the examination system at Key Stages 3 and 4 by the examination boards that takes into consideration the needs of some dyslexic pupils and those with learning differences. There can be special arrangements, such as extra time, readers and amanuensis based on individual need. We are regularly asked the following questions by colleagues and parents prior to SATs and GCSE:

- Is my child eligible for extra time?

- Will the school make an application for extra time on my child's behalf?

- Does my child need a statement to get a reader?

The answers to these questions vary, as each application is treated individually. A pupil does not need a Statement of Educational Need for the school to apply to the Board for these special arrangements. However, there must be evidence of need supported by a suitably qualified professional who is recognised by the Board. Not all qualified special needs teachers can give an assessment, as the Board will only recognise certain qualifications obtained from specific universities. Your school will have a current list of what qualifications a teacher assessor will need and what is acceptable or not. If your school does not have a suitably qualified person then your local education authority's educational psychologist should make an assessment of need and support the application if appropriate. This should be carried out in the two years prior to the examination. The criteria for special arrangements are strictly objective and based on individual application to the Board, which must be made through the school's examination officer and SENCO. The message here is to notify the relevant staff at the school in plenty of time and talk it over with them if there are any concerns that your child or pupil may be dyslexic.

Revision techniques

The aim is: 'Revising using the maximum efficiency with the minimum of effort.' Revision is another word for reviewing. It is the process of rereading and learning essays, coursework, class notes, text books, handouts etc. in order to understand and remember what has been taught. The way forward is to be organised, know your learning style and use it to adopt techniques to learn efficiently. In its simplest form it is knowing yourself and how you learn best.

Organisation

As previously stated, preparing for exams is a long-term process. If pupils have had the experience and practice of learning in a multisensory way, their notes will be dyslexia-friendly. We hope that when our pupils sit down and plan their revision time, they are not phased by the enormity of what is to be done. When pupils are faced with a variety of accessible materials from which to revise, that have been personalised throughout their course, there should be no last minute panic by either the teacher or the pupil. Expectations about what has to be achieved and ways to achieve it have become automatic. They are faced with their own symbols, their own colours and notes that suit their preferred learning style. In this situation both the teacher and the pupil feel secure that the material with which they are familiar is available to revise from.

Time

Use time sensibly. It is a precious commodity. No one wants to spend their lives revising and not having any time left for socialising and leisure activities. The aim is for quality revision time achieving maximum efficiency from minimum effort. Here are some techniques to help to achieve this:

- Make a plan of what has to be done and build up a revision programme from it.

- Keep a time chart for a week to work out how long is spent eating, sleeping, socialising, watching TV, travelling to school, revision. Be honest!

- Build in breaks to the programme – revision periods should not be longer than one hour to be efficient and effective. Go for a short walk in between.

- Make sure there is enough time to revise – be realistic.

- Know the date and time of the exams.

- Know what needs to be learned for each exam.

- Take the right equipment for each exam.

- Try to study in the same place, away from distractions.

- Be comfortable when revising.

- Use a multisensory approach and preferred learning style.

- Use Mind maps© when possible if they suit your style.

Good learning attitudes and habits do work. With effective revision doors of choice will open up. It is important that individual preferred learning styles are recognised and adopted. A learning style or

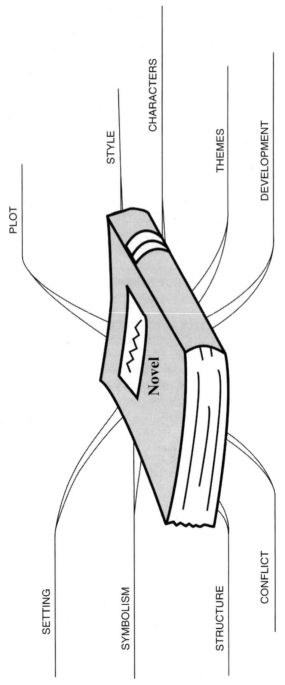

Figure 6.1 Studying Literature Frame

preference is the way information is received and processed by an individual. It is unique to that person and as personal as their fingerprints. Most learners fall into one of three categories – auditory, visual or tactile. Some may have combinations of two and some of three. What is important here is that the learner recognises and uses their preferred method of learning because it is more effective for them. Thus the visual learner will use visual techniques to learn and revise, rather than relying on auditory means, and vice versa. There are many excellent charts and questionnaires available that help to determine the type of learner and his or her preferred learning style.

Mindmapping©

Mindmapping© is the creation of Tony Buzan and is a highly structured and effective technique to use for planning, writing and revision. Tony Buzan's books and videos on Mindmapping© are excellent and have been used successfully in schools with all pupils for a number of years. It is a technique that organises and structures thoughts, materials and ideas on paper so that the pupil can see the 'big' picture or overview and how the components are interrelated. It does not suit all but we would recommend that it be taught to all pupils so that they can make the choice of whether it is useful to them or not. It relies not on linear learning but on a visual approach that is associated with the right side of the brain. This technique is good for dyslexic learners because it plays to their strengths, saves time, helps memory, uses trigger or key words for main points and is a form of revision. In other words, it achieves the aim we started with: 'Revising using the maximum efficiency with the minimum of effort.'

Chapter 7

Conclusion and Summary

This book has been written as a practical aid to help pupils, their parents and mainstream teachers to overcome some of the barriers dyslexia can present in the mainstream English classroom. It is not intended to be an academic reference book. Our ideas are based on real day-to-day teaching experience and the way we believe dyslexic learners should be supported in the secondary school. We are concerned with the whole child and therefore we have stressed throughout the book ways in which dyslexic pupils can become confident and happy learners. Our approaches and methods ensure that the anxieties that are sometimes experienced when teaching dyslexic learners for the first time in the mainstream English classroom can be allayed. We aim to provide the confidence to 'have a go' based on what has worked for us. Once staff have taught pupils with dyslexia they see the pupils' strengths and weaknesses for themselves.

'Good dyslexic teaching practice is good teaching practice' (Turner 2001). We have set out clear, simple strategies that are underpinned by a knowledge of what the pupils are up against and suitable ways to manoeuvre through these difficulties. We believe that good teaching takes account of learning styles, scaffolds development, is multisensory and is success driven. In our experience these straightforward methods support all pupils.

We hope that this book will be a resource to support successful partnerships between staff, pupils and parents, providing a structure that outlines good practice and gives helpful ideas for ways forward.

We feel that we have provided a framework to support dialogue between the 'team members'. We make it clear in meetings that parents, pupils and teachers all have an equal and valuable contribution and part to play in the team. At the heart of partnership is a shared goal in maximising learning potential, ameliorating learning difficulties and raising self-esteem.

The book aims to dispel the myth that only specialist dyslexia teachers can teach dyslexic pupils successfully in the mainstream classroom. Armed with some of the ideas we have put forward we hope that the reader has gained confidence to deliver the full English curriculum in a dyslexia-friendly way. With approximately 10 per cent of the population being dyslexic, the reality is that the majority of dyslexic pupils are taught in mainstream classrooms by non-specialist teachers. We believe that when pupils are taught by English specialists who are equipped with the knowledge of how to deliver the English curriculum in this dyslexia-friendly way, then pupils have the best of both worlds. They have a teacher who removes the obstacles of dyslexia and who is passionate and knowledgeable about their subject area. For pupils who are severely dyslexic and who need an intensive programme specifically designed to meet their emerging literacy needs there should be some additional complementary provision provided by the SEN department. This should run alongside what is done in the mainstream classroom. For example, at Hawarden School the pupils identified by the county as being in greatest need receive specific programmes of work in a small-group setting designed to ameliorate severe reading, writing and spelling difficulties. These pupils are then taught English language and literature by English specialists in their mainstream classroom.

The teacher's job is therefore threefold: to encourage the continued development and practice of good coping strategies; to remove obstacles that prevent access to the subject; and, most importantly, to motivate and generate a willingness to want to analyse, study, read and write in English lessons.

Our vision is that the richness of English should be accessible to all pupils. Once teachers are willing to appreciate this, they become motivated to manoeuvre around weak literacy skills in order to provide access to literature and language. Just because a pupil reads slowly and laboriously, writes and spells in a non-accurate way, doesn't mean that they can't enjoy and be successful in English.

'Can I really get a C, can I, Miss?'

'Who would have thought I would be sitting A levels?'

Two real quotes from two real pupils. They are the reason we have given time to this project. We have seen success for dyslexic learners in GCSEs, A levels and at degree level. However, this is not the only point. These young people are motivated, confident and happy. They have doors of choice open to them. They believe in themselves and have high expectations. This optimism is what we hope to convey to our readers. Being dyslexic means you learn and process information in a way that is different from the norm. As teachers we need to find that way and guide our pupils down it so that they also have doors of choice open to them and achieve their undoubted potential.

Pointers for staff development

Unravelling the pupil from the learning difference is the first step towards successful inclusion. The following pointers set out what is positive and good about being dyslexic, and what teachers need to remember about their dyslexic pupils.

- Dyslexic pupils can do well in English.

- Dyslexic pupils are entitled to inclusion in all aspects of English.

- Harness the power of oracy.

- Dyslexic pupils have very good thinking skills.

- There are many tools available to make school a fairer place for dyslexic learners.

- Use a multisensory approach.

- Be aware that stress and fatigue can be a real problem for dyslexic pupils.

- Dyslexic learners have to work harder.

- Dyslexia can't be cured like chickenpox! It can get easier as you get older and if you are taught coping strategies.

- Self-esteem and confidence make all the difference.

- Technology enhances learning.

- Empower dyslexic pupils to learn how to learn.

- Recognise learning styles – your own and your pupils'.

- Accept alternative ways of presenting work.

- Teaching dyslexic pupils can be extremely rewarding.

- Dyslexia is an explanation, not an excuse.

- Remember what is gained by being dyslexic.

- Use successful dyslexic people as role models. Start a 'Wall of Fame': Churchill, Einstein, Edison . . . Don't forget to use local successes and past pupils.

- Techniques that benefit dyslexic pupils benefit all pupils.

Resources

There are many resources available on the market to help dyslexic pupils. We have included a small selection of those we have used and found helpful.

Tracking Exercises in High Frequency Words and Sentences. Anne Arbour Publishers Ltd, PO Box 1, Belford, Northumberland.

Augur, J. and Briggs, S. *The Hickey Multisensory Teaching System.* London: Whurr.

Cowdery, L. *The Spelling Notebook.* Wrexham: Frondeg Hall Technical Publishing.

Moseley, D. *ACE Spelling Dictionary.* Cambridge: LDA.

Hornsby, B. *Alpha to Omega.* Oxford: Heinemann.

Cowling, K. and Cowling, H. *Toe by Toe.* 8 Green Road, Basildon, West Yorkshire.

Stile Phonic and Spelling Books 1–14. Cambridge: LDA.

Stile Comprehension Books 1–12. Cambridge: LDA.

Stile Grammar and Punctuation Books 1–12. Cambridge: LDA.

Page, P. and Pettit, M. (eds) *Livewire.* London: The Basic Skills Agency.

Baker, J., Constant, C. and Kitchen, D. *Access English.* Oxford: Heinemann.

The Somerset Talking Computer Project Learning Materials. Harlow: Longman.

Walton, J. *The Golden Key Spelling Rules!* Golden Key Publications, 28 Mandeville Road, Hertford.

Walker, M. A. *Resource Pack for Tutors of Students with SpLd.*

ICT

Wordshark 3. Whitespace (Tel. 0208 748 5927).

Superspell (CD-ROM). 4Mation, 14 Castle Park Road, Barnstaple, Devon.

Catchup (CD-ROM). Oxford Brookes University (catchup@brookes.ac.uk).

Numbershark (CD-ROM). Whitespace (Tel. 0208 748 5927).

Superspell Assessment (CD-ROM). Hoopers Multimedia, 4Mation, 14 Castle Park Road, Barnstaple, Devon.

I Love Spelling. London: Dorling Kindersley.

Text Help. Lorien Systems.

Word Search Creator. Neptune Computer Technology.

Via Voice Executive. IBM.

Blyton, E. *The Famous Five*. Systems Integrated Research (SIR) Talking Books.

Success Builders GCSE Chemistry, Biology, Physics, English, Maths. The Learning Company.

GCSE Literature: Orwell, G. *Animal Farm*. Harlow: Longman (school version).

GCSE Literature: Shakespeare. *Macbeth*. Harlow: Longman (school version).

Type to Learn. Iona Software.

Studywiz. Softgram AB.

Bibliography

Augur, J. and Briggs, S. (1993) *The Hickey Multisensory Language Course*. London: Whurr.

Buzan, A. (1993) *The Mind-map Book – Radiant Thinking*. London: BBC.

Cooke, A. (1993) *Tackling Dyslexia the Bangor Way*. London: Whurr.

Hulme, C. and Snowling, M. (eds) (1994) *Reading Development and Dyslexia*. London: Whurr.

Hulme, C. and Snowling, M. (eds) (1997) *Dyslexia: Biology, Cognition and Intervention*. London: Whurr.

Miles, E. (1993) *The Bangor Dyslexia Teaching System*, 2nd edn. London: Whurr.

Moseley, D. (1995) *ACE Spelling Dictionary*, 7th edn. Wisbech: LDA.

Payne, T. and Turner, E. (1999) *Dyslexia: A Parents' and Teachers' Guide*. Clevedon: Multilingual Matters Ltd.

Peer, L. (1999) 'What is dyslexia?', in *The Dyslexia Handbook 61*. Reading: British Dyslexia Association.

Pollock, J. and Waller, E. (1994) *Day to Day Dyslexia in the English Classroom*. London: Routledge.

Pumfrey, P. D. and Reason, R. (1998) *Specific Learning Difficulties (Dyslexia): Challenges and Responses*. London: Routledge.

Reid, G. (2003) *Dyslexia: A Practitioner's Handbook*, 3rd edn. Chichester: Wiley.

Rollason, H. (2000) *Life's too Short*. London: Hodder & Stoughton.

Snowling, M. and Thomson, M. (eds) (1991) *Dyslexia: Integrating Theory and Practice*. London: Whurr.

Thomson, M. and Watkins, E. J. (1993) *Dyslexia: A Teaching Handbook*. London: Whurr.

Turner, E. (2001) 'Dyslexia and English', in L. Peer and G. Reid (eds), *Dyslexia: Successful Inclusion in the Secondary School*. London: David Fulton Publishers.

West, T. G. (1991) *In the Mind's Eye*. New York: Prometheus.

Westwood, P. (1997) *Commonsense Methods for Children with Special Needs*, 3rd edn. London: Routledge.